Geriatric   Nursing

Modern Practical Nursing Series

13

Geriatric Nursing

Bernard Isaacs, M.D., F.R.C.P. (Glasg.), M.R.C.P. (Edin.)

Consultant Physician, Department of Geriatric Medicine, Glasgow Royal Infirmary.

E. M. Burns, R.G.N., S.C.M., Nursing Admin. (Hospital) Certificate

formerly Nursing Officer, Lightburn Hospital, Glasgow. presently Senior Nursing Officer, Canniesburn Hospital, Glasgow.

Thomas Gracie, S.R.N., R.N.T., B.T.A.

Nurse Tutor, Glasgow Royal Infirmary.

WILLIAM HEINEMANN MEDICAL BOOKS LIMITED
LONDON

*Dedicated to many
people — past and present —
in Lightburn Hospital.
They have taught
us much that we
know.*

First Published 1973
© E. M. Burns, Bernard Isaacs and Thomas Gracie 1973
ISBN 0 433 12540 3

Typeset by H Charlesworth & Co Ltd, Huddersfield
Printed in Great Britain
by The Redwood Press Ltd, Trowbridge, Wiltshire

CONTENTS

FOREWORD

We have written this book to help those who are concerned in the care of old people. It is designed primarily for nurses, but we hope that it will prove helpful also to other professional people working with the elderly sick, and to those many devoted relatives, neighbours, friends and voluntary workers who care for ill old people at home.

We express our gratitude to our colleagues in Lightburn Hospital — nurses, physiotherapists, occupational therapists, speech therapists, medical social workers and doctors — for their practical help and advice in the preparation of the text; to Yvonne Neville for her illustrations; and to Isobel Marshall for the great trouble which she has taken in the compilation of the text.

B.I.
T.G.
E.B.

1
About Old People

Geriatrics is concerned with the care of old people.

The era in which we live, the second half of the twentieth century, differs from any previous period of history in that the population contains far more old people than ever before. Even in biblical times it was known that 'the days of our years are threescore years and ten, or, by reason of special strength fourscore years', but very few people ever attained that age. War, famine, and pestilence destroyed most of the populace in infancy, childhood or early adult life.

Today, two-thirds of the population survive to reach their sixty-fifth birthday, and having done so, they can expect to live for another ten to fifteen years on average.

The very old have numerous financial, social and health needs and this is why so many new services and facilities have been created to help them.

Of course not all old people are ill or alone. Everyone knows old ladies or gentlemen in their nineties who are as fit and vigorous and as mentally alert as ever they were. These are a remarkable group of people who often come from long-lived families and who seem to be made of superior material. We hear of centenarians who read books, watch television, write letters, go for long walks and even remain at work. But these are the exceptions, and for the majority it is common to observe some slowing down of physical and mental vigour in the later years, particularly after the age of 75.

What is the reason for this slowing down? It is not old age itself, because old age is not a disease. Just because people are ill *when* they are old one should not conclude that they are ill *because* they are old. Certainly old age is a time of life when illness is common and there are two reasons for this. Firstly, many diseases such as cataract, deafness, hardening of the arteries and cancer become more common with advancing age. Secondly, the old person's body frequently bears the scars of previous disease or injury; for example a man who damaged his knee while playing football at the age of twenty may have arthritis in that same knee when he is eighty; or someone who had a coronary thrombosis at sixty but recovered and returned to work may have heart failure when he is seventy. Because of these two processes, an increased likelihood of certain new diseases, and the accumulation of previous diseases we find that, with advancing age, an increasing proportion of the elderly population are likely to suffer from physical disability.

Among the elderly too, there is much mental disability. This can be of two kinds. On the one hand there is the sadness, apathy, irritability, loneliness, bereavement, loss of contact with family and friends and loss of any definite role in society. We group these as *emotional* changes. On the other hand are the intellectual changes which manifest themselves as loss of memory, impaired powers of concentration and difficulty in learning. Again these changes occur only to some old people. Among the youngest geriatric patients are those over the age of ninety who often remain remarkably alert. No more is depression a feature of all old people. Many of those who seem to have most to be depressed about, remain wonderfully cheerful, never complain about their lot and seem anxious only to help others. Many of these are deeply religious people. But there remain many others who are seriously handicapped in their advanced years by failure of their mental powers.

No one working with old people can ignore the social aspects of their patients. What kind of people are they? What is their life like outside hospital? Who is there to care for them? A person who is aged eighty in 1970 would have been born in 1890 near the end of Queen Victoria's reign, probably of a large family. Unless his parents were well-to-do, he would have left school at the age of twelve and started to work a ten- or twelve-hour day, six days a week for which he would earn perhaps five or ten shillings (25 or 50 new pence) a week. A girl only a little older might have entered domestic service and worked as a maid in a big house from 6 am to 9 pm with perhaps an hour or two off during the day, two hours on Sunday to go to church and a Sunday afternoon and evening once a month to visit her parents. For this she earned £1 a month and her 'keep'. The men joined the Army in the First World War and lived through the appalling battles in France and Flanders. Often they came back to a life of national poverty, unemployment and depression when fit men roamed the streets desperate for work to give

4

them self respect as well as bread and to avoid the humiliation of the 'dole'. Just when things began to get a little better the Second World War came along, with the disruption of family life, and all its terrors and privations.

After the war came slump and confusion again and just when the era of modern affluence was about to begin, it was time for him to retire. Now he has spent fifteen years of his life trying to make ends meet, in the face of ever-rising costs of food, fuel, transport and accommodation. His pension is a few pounds a week and he sees youngsters, a quarter of his age earning four or five times as much.

It is always fascinating to hear old people tell the story of their past and present lives.

The Patient's Family

The most important question is what immediate family does the patient have? In most geriatric units it will be found that only half the men and probably less than a quarter of the women are married. The difference between the sexes is because men tend to be older than their wives and thus to be the first to die and also because men do not, for some unknown reason, live as long as women. A majority of geriatric patients are widowed or unmarried and almost one third of them live alone. Those who live alone are less ill than those who live with a family because having no one to look after them they come into hospital at an earlier stage of their disease. But not all who live alone are lonely and isolated. Many of them do so by choice, preferring to have a home of their own to going to live with relatives; but they are visited frequently and are well looked after. Many of those who live with their married children are very content, but others find that there are great strains in living in a three-generation household where the different needs of the three generations have to be met at once. Many other geriatric patients have no children or their children have emigrated. Perhaps the most tragic cases of all are the recently bereaved, especially the widowers who find that the loss of the life partner coming at a time of physical frailty and after the establishment of life-long habits, is a change to which they are unable to adapt themselves.

Contrary to widely held beliefs, wilful neglect of old people by their relatives very rarely occurs. In those few cases of apparent neglect which are seen there is almost always, on careful enquiry, a good reason for the situation. This usually turns out to be either that the daughter, who may herself be in her fifties or sixties is harassed out of her mind by many other cares; or that the patient is an impossible person to live with — perhaps an alcoholic or a criminal or just a domineering inter-fering old busy body who makes everyone's life a misery.

It is easy to be sentimental about old people. There are many sweet old people but there are also a lot of selfish old people just as there are sweet and selfish young people.

Neglect is uncommon but long and selfless devotion is very common. Many a son or daughter or neighbour or more distant relative is prepared to make a great personal sacrifice in order to help an old person in need. This fact is emphasized because of the importance of a nurse giving every consideration to the relatives of their patients.

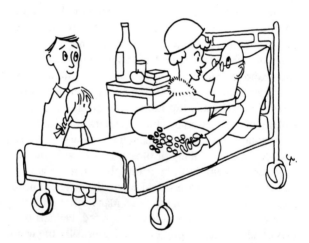

Most relatives are extremely co-operative; some can be a little trying at times; but these are the ones whose whole lives have been wrapped up in caring for their old kinsfolk.

2
The Geriatric Unit

Geriatric units are here to stay. In future more and more nurses will work in them. The need for these units is not created as some would have us believe, by any lessening of a sense of family responsibility. The need is there because, thanks to modern medicine and altered social conditions we have more people than ever before surviving into advanced old age, needing skilled treatment and in many cases having no one available to help them. Where there are families and where their difficulties are properly understood and respected, they will collaborate most willingly in the efforts of the hospital team to provide better care for the old ill people.

In the United Kingdom in 1970 there were almost 200 geriatric units. When did these come about and how do they differ from ordinary medical units?

History of Geriatrics

The majority of geriatric units in the United Kingdom have developed since 1948 when the National Health Service was introduced. How were ill old people looked after before then? Many were cared for at home, just as many still are today, with the difference that in some cases in the past it was the accepted thing that a daughter should remain unmarried and untrained for employment and should stay at home for years on end in order to look after an ageing parent — something that is not often done today. Some old people were treated in general hospitals, as is still the practice, but many others gained admission to special wards for the chronic sick. Some of these were situated in hospitals, some in places called 'Homes for incurables'. Many other chronic sick wards were located in *'Poor Houses', built in the middle of the nineteenth century,* to house the needy and the homeless and subsequently used also for nursing the old and the helpless.

7

In a great majority of these places patients received only a bare minimum of medical and nursing attention. They were kept in bed for years on end, long after they had recovered from the disease for which

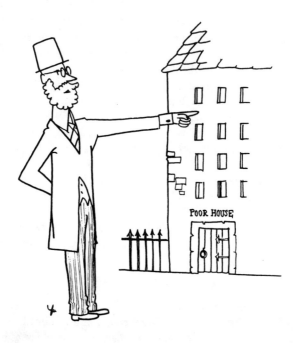

they had been admitted, without any real attempt being made to find out what was wrong with them or to treat them, while the standard of basic nursing care they received — food, warmth, cleanliness, space and facilities was appallingly low.

There were of course exceptions — places where ill old people were cared for with kindness and compassion and in good conditions — but they were unusual. Nevertheless it was in these horrible chronic wards in the 1930's that pioneers of geriatrics began their work. When the National Health Service began in 1948 the hospitals of the chronic sick became the responsibility of the Regional Hospital Boards, and the standards of equipment and treatment began to rise. Many of the best known geriatric units in the country originated in old workhouses. In the 1950's following upon the introduction of antibiotics and improvement in public health there was a reduction in the need of hospital beds for tuberculosis and infective diseases and many such wards were converted into geriatric units. In the 1960's 'purpose built' geriatric units began to appear all over the country and from the 1970's on all the new district general hospitals are to contain a geriatric unit.

So the Geriatric Unit is now part of The Community.

Organisation of a Geriatric unit

The modern geriatric unit has ten clearly defined aims:

1 to advise on the management of old people at home,

2 to admit ill old people from their homes, from old people's homes or from other hospital units,

3 to find out exactly what is wrong with them,

4 to give them appropriate medical and nursing care,

5 to restore as much as possible their ability to live a full and independent life,

6 to study their social and psychological needs,

7 to encourage them to return to an independent life at home,

8 to continue to support and help them after they leave hospital,

9 to provide a good environment and appropriate care for those who are unfit to leave hospital,

10 to enlighten and support relatives; to maintain close contact with organizations which help old people.

In practice this is how these aims are achieved. Every geriatric unit has an *office* which can be contacted by general practitioners and hospital doctors seeking help for an elderly patient.

1 1 A *doctor* from the geriatric unit then arranges to see the patient. Either the doctor visits the patient in his own home, where he sees for himself the whole problem, including the housing situation, the help available, the attitude of relatives and so on

2   Or he brings the patient up to the Out Patient Department for full examination and investigation.

He may then decide either:

1   To admit the patient
2   To treat him as an outpatient or day patient
3   To refer him to some other unit such as an orthopaedic or psychiatric department
4   To advise the general practitioner on home treatment

This last may include the provision of some special service at home, like physiotherapy, the District Nurse or Meals on Wheels.

Most geriatric departments have an admission unit. Here the doctors establish the diagnosis and start treatment. The next stage is a rehabilitation unit (sometimes combined with the admission unit, sometimes separate) where the emphasis is on restoring the patient to functional independence.

1 Teaching him to get into and out of bed
2 Teaching him to get on and off a chair
3 Teaching him to get on and off a commode
4 Teaching him to get on and off a toilet
5 Teaching him to walk
6 Teaching him to climb stairs
7 Teaching him to wash, shave, dress
8 Teaching him to have a bath
9 Teaching him to prepare simple meals in the kitchen
10 Teaching him to perform basic domestic tasks

There are also wards for those patients who have failed to benefit sufficiently from rehabilitation and require to remain in hospital. In addition to these, some departments have wards for special purposes eg for orthopaedic, psychogeriatric or stroke cases.

Another feature of many geriatric departments is a Day Hospital—a unit where patients come in the morning and go home at night. The Day Hospital is open for five days a week, and individual patients attend once or twice a week, sometimes more often, sometimes less. At the

Day Hospital they have medical and nursing treatment, but the emphasis is on rehabilitation and diversionary activities.

Most geriatric departments also have a follow-up service for patients to be seen for supervision after discharge, either at home or at the out-patient clinic or Day Hospital.

A nurse in a geriatric unit is closely concerned, not only with caring for ill patients but also with all aspects of the patient's rehabilitation. She can be of very great help in encouraging the patient towards independence and she can at the same time listen to and learn from the patient, who is ready to confide in her, all the problems and anxieties that worry him.

The Geriatric Team

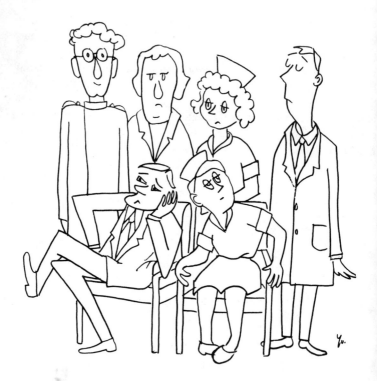

In a geriatric unit

1 Doctors
2 Nurses
3 Physiotherapists
4 Occupational therapists
5 Social Workers
6 Chaplains

form a team of people, each with some special knowledge, who share their ideas and experience in order to give better treatment to the patient.

In most units some form of Case Conference is held every week at which the progress of each patient is discussed; and there is no better way of learning from one another. Some units arrange for nurses to work with the physiotherapist and occupational therapist so as to learn at first hand what is done for the patient. In many departments too, people come into hospital from the community to discuss patient care.

1 District nurses
2 Health visitors
3 Social workers for local authorities
4 Family doctors
5 Members of voluntary organisations

Some departments make arrangements for their nurses to:

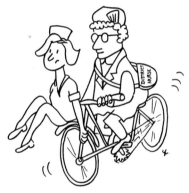

1 accompany the District Nurse on her rounds,
2 go out with the Meals-on-Wheels service,
3 visit Old Peoples Homes and clubs.

The real feature of nursing in a geriatric unit is the nurse's full involvement in every aspect of the patient's case. Given this outlook and the opportunity to work in this way very few nurses find work in a geriatric unit depressing; the great majority derive much satisfaction from knowing that they are really helping to restore ill old people to the enjoyment of independent living in their own homes; or, if that is not possible, are providing them with a life of contentment in hospital.

3
Physical and Mental Changes in Old Age

In this chapter an account will be given of some of the more frequently encountered diseases of old people. The conditions to be described are all so common that any one old person is liable to have more than one disability at a time. For example a patient who takes a stroke may also have heart disease. For his stroke he needs exercise, for his heart disease he needs rest — how is he to be treated? That is a matter for the doctor to judge very carefully. Or a patient with Parkinson's disease may lose his eyesight. If he had either disability alone it would be straightforward to rehabilitate him, with both together this becomes a very difficult task. Another feature of illness in old people is the way in which physical, mental and social factors may interact. For example an old man's wife dies. He lives alone and has no children. He becomes depressed. He makes little effort to shop or cook. He does not go out. He begins to suffer from the effects of malnutrition. He becomes flabby from lack of exercise. One night he falls; he is too weak to rise, he is forced to lie on the floor all night. No one is in the habit of coming to see him, so it may be late next day before he is discovered and brought to hospital as a patient with combined physical, mental and social disability.

Physical changes

There is of course a vast number of diseases from which old people suffer and these are described in medical textbooks. We can group some of the more important ones into a few general categories:

Cardio-respiratory	Nutritional
Locomotor	Disturbance of bladder and bowel
Neurological	Malignant
Special senses	Others

Only a very short outline of these will be given here and the interested reader should consult a textbook for detailed descriptions.

Cardio-respiratory Diseases

Cardio-respiratory diseases include numerous conditions affecting the heart or lungs. Some of these, like chronic bronchitis may have been present for many years; others, like coronary artery disease, may come on in middle or late life; others again, like pneumonia may be acute illnesses. These conditions usually cause breathlessness on exertion or at rest, ease of fatigue and weakness; while some of the diseases may cause coughing, spitting, hoarseness, pain in the chest on breathing or on exertion, and swelling of the ankles. Diseases of this group are very common, but often a great deal can be done to help the sufferers.

Locomotor Disorders

Locomotor disorders are those conditions which prevent the patient from getting about. The commonest of these are diseases of the joints, like osteoarthritis and rheumatoid arthritis, and conditions causing paralysis of muscles (which will be described in the next section). Also included in this group are injuries like fractures of the neck of the femur, amputations and conditions causing muscle weakness. Patients with arthritis may be so severely crippled that they are confined to bed or to a wheelchair; or they may have limited ability to get about in the house but are unable to climb stairs or to walk out of doors. They may be liable to falls. Often they suffer pain and stiffness in the joints, and sometimes their limbs are twisted into abnormal shapes. In this group too, it is often possible to help patients a great deal by medical treatment, by physiotherapy and sometimes even by surgery.

Neurological Disorders

Neurological disorders include diseases of the brain, the spinal cord or the nerves, which cause paralysis, loss of sensation or loss of ability to speak. The commonest neurological disorder in geriatric patients is a stroke, which occurs with increasing frequency from about the age of fifty onwards and which usually causes paralysis of one side of the body and sometimes loss of speech as well. Although this is a very crippling disease very good results can be obtained with modern treatment.

15

Another common neurological disease
is *Parkinson's Disease* which *affects the
gait* and balance and which may cause falls.

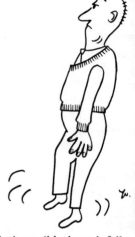

There are many other diseases which cause dizziness, 'blackouts', falls,
fits, pain or paralysis and which require careful assessment and treatment.

The Special Senses
The special senses include vision, hearing, smell and taste. Blindness is a
dreadful handicap at any age, but is particularly tragic in the old
person, who finds it so difficult to adapt himself to a world of darkness.
Yet some of the diseases which threaten the old person's sight can be
treated, and even those patients who become blind can be taught to live
with their handicap. Deafness is perhaps an even greater tragedy, for the
deaf person becomes cut off from contact with his fellowmen and deaf
old people are often very depressed or even paranoid. Many conceal
their disability and are thought to be stupid or irritable rather than deaf.
Others are reluctant to wear hearing aids which make them feel self-
conscious and they do not like the distortion which the aid causes. They
should be encouraged to persevere. The deaf should always be treated
with the utmost tact and consideration. Deafness is discussed in more
detail in chapter 6. Many old people lose their sense of taste and thus
lose their enjoyment of food. The sense of smell is also frequently lost,
and this can have the serious effect of gassing accidents.

Nutritional Disturbance

Nutritional distrubances found in old people include deficiencies of protein, calcium, of iron and vitamins notably C and D. The main cause of these deficiencies is apathy, usually in patients living alone who cannot be bothered preparing proper meals. These deficiencies lead to weakness, softening of the bones, weakening of the muscles and susceptibility to infection. Another nutritional disturbance is *obesity*, due to eating too much of the wrong kind of food. This is bad in itself, and is also often associated with other conditions such as heart disease, diabetes and arthritis.

Bladder and Bowel Disturbances

Bladder and bowel disturbances include frequency, urgency and precipitancy of micturition, which means that the patient has to pass water much more often than normal; that, as soon as he feels the need it becomes very strong; and that he is unable to restrain himself unless he has an immediate opportunity to pass water. This symptom is sometimes accompanied by pain on passing water. Retention of urine means that the patient is unable to pass urine at all or he has a 'stoppage' of his water and needs a catheter or other form of help. Incontinence of urine is often, but not always, associated with mental impairment. Constipation is the commonest bowel trouble. It is frequent in old people and can be very troublesome indeed, occasionally reaching such a severe degree that the lower bowel becomes blocked with a mass of faeces. These conditions are described in more detail in chapters 10 and 11. A number of other diseases like diverticulitis and haemorrhoids can cause bowel upsets and bleeding from the bowel.

Malignant Diseases

Malignant disease means cancer, which is commonly found in old people. Cancer is a dreaded disease because so often it destroys a person in the prime of life and because its course can be protracted and painful. In general cancer is a milder disease in old age. It may be present for months or years without causing any symptoms, or it may be responsible only for a general feeling of weakness that is ascribed inevitably to 'old age'. Many old people with cancer never know they have had it and die quietly in their sleep. Other cases can be treated with excellent results even in very old age. There are of course other less happy cases but there is no reason in old people (or indeed in people of any age) to think of the diagnosis of cancer as meaning a sentence of lingering painful death (see further reading list page 183).

Other Diseases

Other diseases include anaemia, gland troubles, digestive upsets, kidney diseases and so on. Old people in geriatric units are usually very thoroughly investigated because of the likelihood of finding several different diseases, some if not all of which can be successfully treated.

Mental Changes

The words most often used to describe mental changes in old people are *dementia* and *confusion*. These are quite different things.

Dementia

Dementia is the name given to a group of diseases in which brain cells are destroyed by degeneration, by loss of their blood supply or by some other cause. As a result the patient is permanently incapable of performing tasks which require memory, or concentration or learning power, although he may cope with simple and familiar routines fairly well.

Confusion

Confusion is a temporary state of mind which affects people with normal or damaged brains. Usually it is a result of some disturbance outside the brain like a high fever, pneumonia or heart disease which causes a temporary state of bewilderment in which the patient may hold quite erroneous beliefs and may be noisy, restless, agitated and fearful.

A proper understanding of these conditions is essential for successful nursing of the geriatric patient and they are described in more detail in chapter 13.

4
Rehabilitation

Rehabilitation means restoring to the patient the ability to function independently. Rehabilitation demands a mixture of enthusiasm and common sense. The enthusiasm is required to ensure that the patient is made as fit as possible — sometimes even better than he was before the illness. The common sense is necessary so that the treatment is not carried to the extent of exhausting the patient.

The aim of rehabilitation in any given case depends on the patient, the nature of his illness and the kind of home to which he will be returning after hospital treatment. The rehabilitation of a man of fifty with a back injury is a different matter from the rehabilitation of a man of seventy-five with a stroke but in both cases we start by asking the same questions: 'What is this patient unable to do as a result of his illness which he requires to do to enable him to lead a satisfactory life and which it is reasonable to expect him to be able to do?'

Rehabilitation and physiotherapy are not the same thing. The physiotherapist plays a very important role in rehabilitation but so do the doctor, the nurse, the occupational therapist, the speech therapist, the social worker, the relatives — everyone in contact with the patient helps in the return of independence.

In this chapter some of the ways in which the nurse participates in rehabilitation will be described.

Rehabilitation begins the moment the patient is brought into the ward. He may be anxious, frightened and depressed. If he sees a gloomy ward or a glum face or if he is left lying unattended the thought may form in his mind 'I will never come out of this place alive'. A negative despondent attitude by the patient is the greatest single obstacle to rehabilitation. On the other hand a *cheerful welcome,* a word of encouragement, planted at the very beginning of the patient's stay in hospital, *can be the start of a successful programme of rehabilitation.*

The other patients in the ward play a valuable role at this early stage, as the following words of a stroke patient testify: 'When I first came into hospital I was in despair; I was convinced that I would never walk

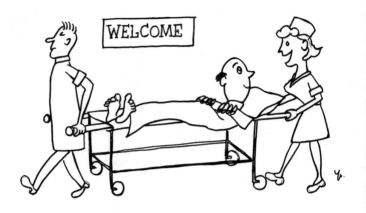

A Cheerful Welcome

again. Then one of the other patients walked over to me and said "Dont worry dear, when I came in here at first I was worse than you and look at me now". Then I said to myself, "If she can do it, so can I" and from that day on I've never looked back'.

Not all patients have the same will power and determination but no good is done by giving them a talking to and telling them that they are not trying to help themselves. Even if this is true, as it sometimes is, the patient only resents being told the unpalatable truth and says to himself for instance, 'It's all very well for her, she has got the use of her legs'. Sometimes a patient does benefit from a talking to but this should be given once properly by a person in authority who is respected by the patient and carefully trained. The nurse's attitude should be one of patience, sympathy and encouragement.

The patient should be trained and encouraged to do things for himself, no matter how simple.

First he is taught:

1 to move himself in bed,
2 to turn to the right and left,
3 to raise his bottom from the bed.

Next he is taught to sit up in bed and to maintain the sitting posture. While he remains in bed he is given exercises to maintain the tone of his muscles and the mobility of his joints Here are a few important but simple exercises which a nurse can do with any patient:

Quadriceps Drill

Quadriceps drill prevents weakness and wasting of the thigh muscles.
The patient lies supine with legs extended.
Nurse places her hand firmly against the sole of each foot in turn to steady it and prevent movement. The patient then alternately tightens and relaxes the quadriceps muscles for a count of five, ten or twenty twice each leg.
The whole exercise should be repeated several times a day.

Prevention of Foot Drop

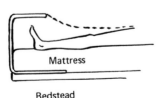

Mattress

Bedstead

Patients with paralysis of legs must have a cage to prevent the bed-clothes pressing the foot downwards. In addition at every opportunity

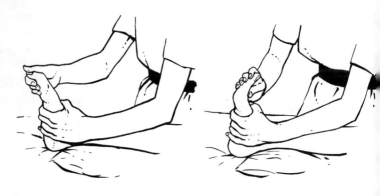

the nurse should correct any tendency for the foot to plantar flex, by pushing the sole into a correct position and holding it there.

Correction of Hand Deformity

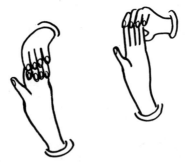

A weak or paralysed hand is in danger of being flexed at the metacarpo-phalangeal and interphalangeal joints and adducted at the thumb, a tendency that is often aggravated by the common but wrong practice of placing a ball in the patient's hand. Instead the nurse should at every opportunity extend the wrist and fingers and abduct the thumb by placing her own hand against the patient's as shown. The patient should also do this for himself.

Mobilization of Shoulders

A weak or paralysed arm tends to drag at the shoulder joint, which may become stiff, painful and 'frozen'. This is prevented by good position, so that the weight of the arm is taken by pillows; and also by putting the arm through its *full* range of movement at every opportunity. The nurse supports the arm by the hand or forearm, brings it across the front of the body (adduction) lifts it up to the side (abduction), then raises it straight above the head (extension) performing all movements slowly and carefully to avoid causing pain.

The Patient Out of Bed

When the patient is ready to get out of bed he should be dressed in his own warm comfortable clothes and shoes, and made to look as smart as possible. This has an immensely important effect on the patient's whole attitude to recovery. Pyjamas, dressing gown and slippers mean invalidism; clothes mean recovery.

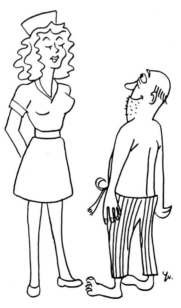

Nurses will quickly become convinced that, although it takes time for patients to dress (or initially to be dressed) in their own clothes, the time is well spent, and in the long run represents time saved, because soon the patient will be able and eager to dress himself. One should not be put off by the thought that he will only mess his clothes. Patients are more likely to make the effort to keep themselves clean and dry when their self respect is restored to them, as no one can feel self respect if they are dressed continually in a dressing gown, nightgown or pyjamas.

Should the Patient be Out of Bed?

Getting patients out of bed is usually desirable but some discretion is required.

There is little point in getting a very frail patient up to sit in a chair if he is nice and comfortable in bed. Some weak patients are tired out with sitting, some slip down on to the floor. No one likes to have to impose any form of restraint on a patient and when there is found to be no way of preventing him from falling out of a chair other than by tying him into it one should ask whether the patient would not be better in bed meantime having muscle-strengthening exercises to prepare him for sitting up.

Chairs

The type of chair is very important. A suitable chair for a geriatric patient should have the following characteristics:

1 The seat should be horizontal and moulded to the shape of the bottom. It should not slope backwards.

2 The front edge should be an inch or two behind the knee

3 The height should be such that the patient can sit comfortably with the soles of the feet flat on the ground and the hips and knees flexed at the correct angle.

4 The patient should be able to sit well back in the chair. This is best achieved by having a gap between the back and the seat of the chair.

5 The back of the chair should be moulded to support the lower dorsal spine.

6 The arms should be padded at elbow height.

A drop arm to give leverage on standing is helpful

7 There should be no cross-member between the front legs so that the patient is free to place the feet well underneath him when attempting to rise

8 The legs should splay out so that the feet are well outside the base of the chair, to give stability.

9 The feet should have rubber stops on them to prevent slipping.

10 The upholstery should be capable of being cleaned simply and there should be no 'crumb traps'.

No chair meets all these requirements but a few in common use have proved generally acceptable.

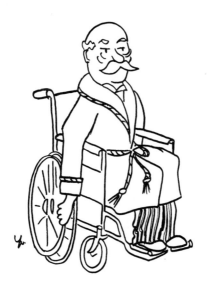

Self-propelled Wheel Chairs

Patients who are able to sit up safely and who have good arm movement should be encouraged to move about in a self-propelled wheel chair. They require some preliminary instruction in its use.

Patients should never sit down in or rise from a wheel chair without first checking that the brakes have been applied. For patients with hemiplegia a special method has been devised to enable them to propel the chair with one arm and one leg. They are taught to hook the normal leg under the paralysed one and to propel the chair by bending and straightening the two legs together using the normal hand to assist in driving and steering. The use of a wheel chair does not delay walking. On the contrary patients learn all the quicker because they are stimulated by moving freely talking to others.

Transferring from Chair to Chair or Commode

Once the patient is able to sit up he needs to learn to *transfer* from bed to chair, *from chair to commode* or wheelchair, from commode back to chair and so back to bed. To illustrate the method, here is how a patient is taught to transfer from chair to chair. If the patient has hemiplegia the chair to which he is going to transfer should be on his normal side. The following description relates to a patient with left hemiplegia; for patients with right hemiplegia the sequence is the opposite.

The nurse helps in this sequence by standing in the angle between chairs or the chair and commode. She can if necessary give support to the patient's right arm.

1 Place the chair in contact with the patient's chair and at right angles to it.
2 The patient rises, supporting himself with his hands on the arms of his own chair.
3 He then reaches over and places his right hand on the right arm of the new chair.
4 Next he swivels his right foot through ninety degrees and slides until his right foot is in front of the new chair.

5 If his left arm is not paralysed he can now relinquish his hold of the
   left arm of the old chair and can grip the left arm of the new chair.
6 He finally draws his left leg into position in front of the new chair
   and he is ready to sit down.

Exactly the same method is used for getting patients on and off a
commode.

Transferring from Chair to Bed

1 The chair is placed at right angles to the side of the bed (right side
   for left hemiplegics) facing the head of the bed and about half way
   along the length.
2 The patient stands, places his right hand on the bed.
3 He rotates his body to face away from the bed and sits down on it.
4 He then hooks his good leg under his weaker one.
5 He lifts it up.
6 He then swings round on his bottom to swing his legs on to the bed.

Bed to Chair

For getting out of bed the chair is placed on the left side of the bed,
again facing the head end. The patient sits up, swings his legs round
with the good one helping its weaker fellow, stands up at the side of the
bed, turns his body, sits down. The nurse gives a little help where it is
needed, but leaves the patient to do as much as he can himself, merely
steadying the chair and being ready to correct any faults which might
cause a fall.

Walking

The main objective of rehabilitation is to enable the patient to walk
safely and independently, and this requires skilled training by the
physiotherapist with whom the nurse should collaborate closely. If
the patient is pronounced by the physiotherapist to be fit to walk on

his own with or without a walking stick then the nurse must see to it that he does walk on his own, and that the appropriate aid is beside him and is correctly used. If he is unable to manage on his own he should be transported in a wheel chair. In between these two groups is a third set of patients who can walk but need the support or supervision of one person. There are three good ways of helping these patients and many bad ways. If the patient cannot be confidently and safely managed in one of these three ways by one person he should be put in a wheel chair and should only walk with the physiotherapist. There is no value in 'walking' a patient between two nurses. The patient does none of the work and derives no benefit. Here are three recommended methods:

Front Support

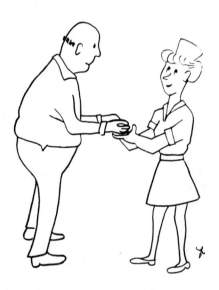

This is suitable for frail and frightened patients, especially those who tend to fall back. The nurse faces the patient and supports him by placing her hands, palm upwards beneath the patient's hand; or in some cases by her forearm under the patient's. The nurse walks backwards step for step with the patient, encouraging him to lean forward. Should the patient show any tendency to fall, the nurse takes a quick step forwards and places her arm round the patient's back to control him.

Side Support

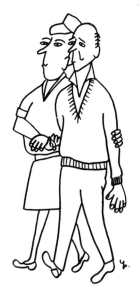

This method is excellent for slightly weak patients and especially for hemiplegics. The nurse walks at the patient's right side and just a little behind him, taking his right hand in her right hand, and placing her left hand behind his back. Sometimes a little pressure on the back from her left hand is required; but usually the hand is just there to catch him should he stagger backwards. She can also very easily move in behind him and catch his body with hers. For a right hemiplegic the nurse of course, walks on the patient's left side.

Back Support
This is moral support only for the almost independent patient who is not yet quite safe. The nurse walks just behind the patient and slightly to the side. Because he cannot see her he is less nervous and less

distracted but she is there waiting just in case he loses balance. She keeps her hands ready at her sides and at the least sign of unsteadiness she steps in behind and corrects his balance.

Walking Aids

Some ambulant patients use walking aids. There is an appropriate aid for each type of patient and it is just as important that the patient should have the right walking aid as that he should be given the right medicine. Patient's walking aids should be labelled with their names and should be kept handy beside the bed or chair. Nurses should check from time to time with the physiotherapist that the correct aid is being used. The following types are needed:

Wooden Walking Stick

This is the simplest type. It is required by patients with mild weakness or arthritis on one side; by those with a slight balance disturbance; and by those with a tendency to grab hold of furniture. The hemiplegic patient takes the stick in the hand opposite to his stroke. The arthritic patient takes the stick in the same side as his arthritis.

The stick has the following characteristics:

a   It is made of stout ash

b   It has a good handle

c   Its height is such that when it is placed upright on the ground and a little in front of the patient his arm is almost straight. When placed beside the patient it should reach his greater trochanter

d   The bottom is covered by a thick rubber ferrule, preferably a crutch-tip, to give a good grip of the ground and to prevent the stick from slipping if it is not placed straight

It is useful for patients who use sticks to have a garment on which the handle of the stick can be hooked when they need to use two hands. There should also be somewhere for the stick to stand safely beside the bed and chair and beside the toilet (eg a spring clip like those used for brushes in a cupboard). Many a patient falls when reaching down to pick his stick off the floor.

Patients should avoid the use of two sticks. They are difficult to handle and almost impossible to put down and there are good alternatives.

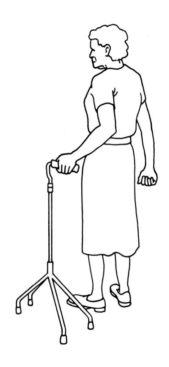

Three or Four-Legged Sticks

These sticks broaden the patient's base and give better support than the ordinary walking stick. They are used especially in the treatment of stroke. They have 'bicycle handle grips', are adjustable for height and size and have good rubber ferrules on all feet and they can stand up by themselves.

Zimmer and other Light Weight Walking Aids

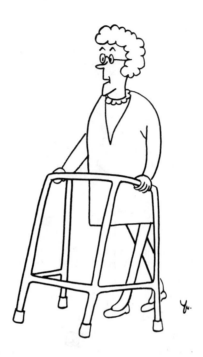

This type of aid is held in both hands. The patient lifts it, places it firmly on all four feet and a foot or two in front of him and takes two paces towards it, then lifts it again and so on.

The aid brings the patient's base forwards and greatly enlarges it, thus giving him greater stability and avoiding any tendency to fall backwards. It is particularly useful for frail people and those with a tendency to fall and to hold on to furniture and for those with arthritis of hips or knees or after a fracture. It helps to take the weight off the joints. It is unsuitable for stroke patients. Since it imparts an unnatural gait pattern, patients should aim to discard it as they improve; but frail old people who would be unable to walk without its help can be helped to remain ambulant by this aid.

The Rollator Walking Aid

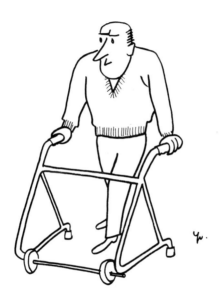

Wheeled aids are in general undesirable because of the danger that they will run away from the patient; but in the Rollator this disadvantage is overcome by the rear legs which are covered with thick rubber pads. The Rollator is pushed in front of the patient like a pram. It gives excellent support and is especially valuable for patients with Parkinson's disease who need such support but who have difficulty in manipulating a 'Zimmer' with their stiff arms. But it needs a smooth floor, it takes up a lot of space, and it is inconvenient to get through a doorway.

Reciprocal Light Weight Walking Aid

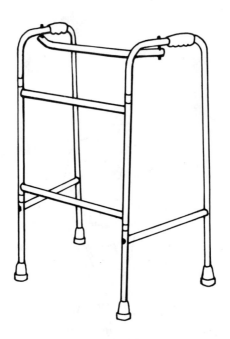

Because each side of the walking frame moves forward alternatively the patient is firmly supported, completely stable, and yet is afforded the maximum freedom of movement.

Helping Hand
People whose mobility is restricted find one of their biggest problems is that of reaching for things they want.

The Helping Hand grips gently and firmly and will grip hard and soft objects.

By using it an elderly housewife can continue to do many of the tasks which would be too difficult for her to manage with restricted mobility.

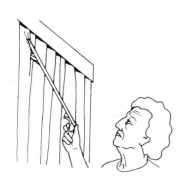

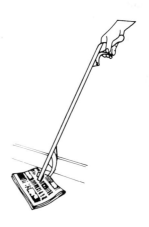

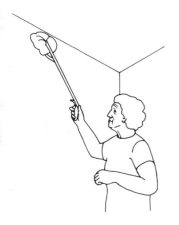

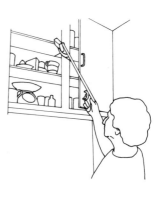

35

These are some of the methods and tools of rehabilitation. There are others to be learned by experience. The nurse who knows what can be done in one sphere of rehabilitation will find solutions to other problems of independent living as they arise. The knowledge will help to form the attitude that no problem is insoluble. By taking thought and making effort patients can be helped to find a way. That is the essence of the art of rehabilitation.

5
The Patient's Day

Any nurse who has been a patient in hospital herself knows how different a day looks from the patient's point of view. Since most patients in geriatric wards are up and dressed the object should be to make their day as interesting and varied and as much like an ordinary day as circumstances allow.

Patients should be wakened as late as ward routine allows and should then use the toilet, wash, dress and have breakfast (not necessarily in that order) as soon as possible. If, as happens in some hospitals patients are wakened very early, given a drink and allowed to go back to sleep their routine will be upset, some will even wake a second time with a wet bed.

Before breakfast they should be toileted, face and hands washed and dentures inserted. Patients able to carry out these activities for themselves should be encouraged to do so. Patients able to dress themselves should be given their clothes, previously laid out by the nurse, in the order they should be put on. The nurse should leave the patient in the position most suitable to him for dressing i.e. on top of the bed or on a chair at the bedside. Patients requiring assistance with dressing can be dressed, if time allows, or sat up in dressing gown and slippers for breakfast.

Less well patients may require to be attended to earlier in the morning, in fact they may well be awake, lying uncomfortably in bed, and welcome attention from the nurses, including changing of wet beds care of pressure areas, changing of position, washing of face and hands and the giving of a drink. Having been made comfortable the patient will settle peacefully until breakfast time.

Breakfast may be served in the dining area, at the bedside or in bed. Those in bed should be propped up, and encouraged to feed themselves with bed table at a convenient height.

After breakfast toileting may again be necessary. Patients already dressed should walk or be assisted to the Day Room. Those still in dressing gowns should be dressed and join the others in the Day Room.

The seating arrangements in the day room influence the pattern of social intercourse. Where the area is small there is little alternative to seating the patients in a row round the wall, when each person can at best manage to converse with two others and then only by craning his neck uncomfortably. Where space allows it is far better to group patients around tables. These should be of a comfortable height, preferably round, with recessed legs so that wheel chairs can be accommodated. This brings each patient face to face with three or four others and facilitates conversation, letter writing and playing games.

In the course of the morning the patient will be given his medicines, any injections or treatments, also a mid-morning drink to ensure an adequate fluid intake.

The patients may visit or be visited by the doctor, the physiotherapist, the occupational therapist or speech therapist. They will have an opportunity to read the daily papers, books or magazines, open mail, play cards and games.

Less well patients must again be attended to. Some may be able to sit up for a short period and this change of position will help to prevent break down of pressure areas.

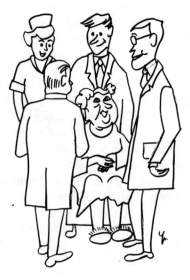

The atmosphere of a geriatric ward is one of cheerful informality. Even for the doctor's round the patients are up and dressed. There is a recognition that the running of the ward is 'patient-centred' rather than 'doctor or nurse centred'.

The patients may require to go to the toilet before lunch and again after lunch. Also after lunch an opportunity should be given for an hour's rest on top of the bed. By early afternoon physiotherapy, speech therapy and occupational therapy treatments will have recommenced and visitors will be beginning to arrive. The medicines will again be given and the afternoon teas. At some time during the day the male patients will be shaved and some patients bathed. By the late afternoon the frailer patients will feel tired and wish to return to bed, visiting the toilet on the way. Quite a proportion of the patients will enjoy having their evening meal in the Dining Area and later having the opportunity to watch television in the Day Room.

Although many things happen during the patient's day there are still long periods when they sit on their chairs staring at the wall. It can be an uphill task to keep them interested and amused, and too much reliance should not be placed on radio and television. Television in particular which has been such a boon to lonely housebound old people, often fails to arouse the geriatric patient from his apathy. Perhaps he does not see the picture or follow the words or understand the situation. It is better to switch the set on specifically for some programme that interests the patients, such as a boxing match, or a family serial, than batter the patient's eyes and ears with non-stop television.

Television sets can be obtained with earphone attachments. These can be a boon in community living.

During the evening the medicines will again be given, treatments carried out and all necessary care given to the bed patients, routines which have continued at regular intervals throughout the day. After the evening meal patients requiring assistance will be prepared for bed. Only patients independent in dressing and toileting can usually remain up into the later part of the evening.

A hot drink is given before the night staff commence the last toilet round of the day. The patients are made comfortable and any necessary sedatives are administered.

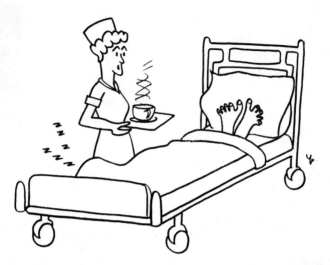

After the sedatives and night drugs have been given the night nurse's main task is toiletting. In addition to dealing with patients who ask for the toilet during the night and with those whose beds have been soiled, she should have a list of patients who are at risk of being incontinent and she should waken these patients once or twice during the night to use the toilet in the hope of preventing incontinence.

Noise is a great enemy of sleep and one which is difficult to eliminate in a hospital. There is no excuse for noisy equipment. A bigger problem is the noisy patient who becomes confused and disturbed at night and keeps the rest of the ward awake. This is a most difficult situation for the night nurse to handle. Sometimes it comes from pain or a need to empty the bladder or bowel, but more often the cause goes deeper and a simple solution does not work. The doctor should be called to investigate the cause and to prescribe treatment and sedation. Often the patient will have to be moved out of the ward area to prevent disturbing other patients, but it is then difficult for the nurses to supervise the noisy patient and the others at the same time, unless additional help can be provided. Usually disturbed patients are put in beds with cot sides, but this may only make matters worse, because they are frightened and resentful of the cot sides. They rattle the sides noisily and try to climb over them. When a patient is determined to get out of bed at night one way to handle the situation is to let him get up, talk to him quietly, give him a cup of tea or a cigarette and hope that he will gradually calm down and return to bed. This may be a counsel of perfection and very disturbed patients require powerful sedation by injection.

Morning comes and the lights are switched on. The night staff go off duty, the day nurses come on. Another day begins for the patients. Will they look forward to it as a day which brings them nearer to discharge to their own homes and families or will they welcome it as bringing them one day nearer death? So much will depend on how the nurses have filled each patient's day.

Visitors

Visiting arrangements in geriatric wards, especially those with proper day rooms and cubicle bedrooms, are usually more flexible than is possible in the general wards. In many units visiting is from 2 pm till 8 pm every day and this poses no great difficulties to the staff. There still tends to be a concentration of visitors in the evenings and at weekends. Visitors must appreciate that if they come in the afternoon, they may have to wait until the patient has had his treatment so it is necessary to have somewhere outside the ward where relatives can wait in comfort and have a cup of tea. Relatives should be encouraged to share the looking after of the patient, for example by feeding and caring for the hair and clothing but they should not walk patients or take them to the toilet without the express permission of the nurse in charge. They must realize that the staff are responsible for any accident which might occur. With long visiting periods conversation sometimes runs dry so relatives should be encouraged to bring in cards and games to play with the patients. Some patients have no visitors, and the nurse should encourage other patient's visitors or voluntary workers to include them in their conversations and activities. Visitors should be put in touch with the physiotherapist, occupational therapist and speech therapist to discuss with them the management of the patient after discharge. Patients can become exhausted by excessive visiting and they can be embarrassed in the visitors presence to ask for the toilet. Some

Voluntary Helpers can —

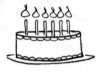

Celebrate Birthdays

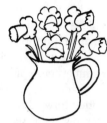

Arrange Flowers

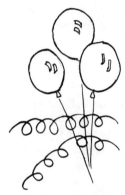

Decorate Wards

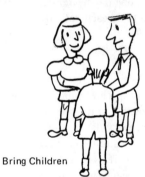

Bring Children

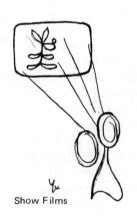

Show Films

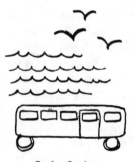
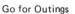

Go for Outings

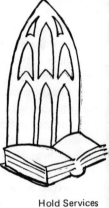

Hold Services

visitors are over generous with food and may have to be advised against giving the patients too much to eat.

Any change in the established pattern of the hospital day is welcomed by the patients. A birthday party, a Women's Guild meeting, a visit from a group of young folk or adults to sing and entertain help to make each day different.

Opportunities to meet patients from other wards at film shows, socials, church services and outings widen horizons from the confines of the ward.

Voluntary helpers can be of great assistance in such activities as well as in the more accepted ways of running trolley shops, library trolleys and providing tea for visitors.

Knowledge of Patients — Recording

The nurse requires to have a detailed knowledge of the patient's abilities otherwise she may leave a patient to dress herself who is not capable of doing so. On the contrary she may dress someone who can dress himself. The night staff, and equally the part time staff are more likely to make this kind of error than are the day staff, because they have not the same opportunity for observing the patient. It is therefore important to have a system of communication which ensures that all nurses know the capabilities of their patients.

The practical way of doing this is by the report, but in a large busy ward with rapidly changing staff and patients it is not always possible to ensure that every nurse learns all details about every patient in this way. One way of classifying the patient's abilities is of coding the instruction required; but the system must be simple if it is to be understood and used properly. Each ward will work out the routine that it finds most suitable, but here are some suggested ways of achieving communication:

The Visible File

On this system each patient's name is written on a card which is inserted in a slit in the visible file. The card can have columns for dressing, feeding, toilet and so on, in which are recorded such categories as 'independent' or 'needs help'. The cards can be checked each week and whenever a change occurs in a patient. The nurse coming on duty should read over the file to see what help each patient requires.

Name	Washing	Toilet	Condition of Skin	Treatment	Dressing	Feeding	Mobility

Another system is to draw attention to any special situation by the use of coloured markers; for example it can be arranged that a red marker inserted in the Kardex means that that patient requires to be dressed and the nurse sees at a glance where the help is needed.

Wall Chart
A board is erected on the wall of the treatment room or other suitable point on which the names of the patients are recorded. Coloured markers are used to signify whether the patient is ambulant, incontinent, is in need of help when feeding, and so on. A space at the bottom of the board explains the markers. This chart must be kept regularly up-to-date.

The amount of information should be limited to three or four items per patient so as to prevent bewildering the nurse.

At the Bedside
Markers or instructions can be attached to the patient's bed where their impact is immediate.

In addition to these routine matters, some patients have temporary special needs eg 'Push fluids' — 'nothing by mouth' 'keep all urine' etc. This will be recorded in the nursing report and the patient himself should be advised, but additionally a blackboard in the treatment room or sluice room can be used. Special cards can be attached to the patient's bed. Another idea is to use one coloured marker on the visible file or wall chart to indicate a special need not otherwise specified and this draws the nurse's attention to the latest entry on the nursing report.

Record of Frequency of Turning

WARD _____ SURNAMES _____ FIRST NAMES _____

FREQUENCY OF TURNING
2 HOURLY _____
4 HOURLY _____
OTHER _____

Date	Time	Position	State of Pressure Sores and Pressure Points when turned	Signature

6
Communication

Throughout every sphere of organized human life the importance of communication is recognised. It has become the habit to attribute everything that goes wrong from strikes to divorces to defects of communication. Particularly the geriatric patient is vulnerable to faulty communication and the nurse as the person to whom he is most likely to wish to communicate in the first place, has a special need to understand the difficulties which face the patient.

Defects of communication may be due to

1 Sensory deprivation
2 Intellectual impairment
3 Social limitations
4 Organizational errors
5 Any combination of these

Sensory Deprivation

This includes deafness and blindness.

Deafness

A hearing defect is one of the commonest and one of the unhappiest reasons for lack of communication. Deafness is very common in old people, especially in those who have had noisy jobs such as boilermaker or pneumatic drillers. The patients have particular difficulty in hearing high-pitched sounds but may hear sounds of lower pitch quite well. The importance of this is that in human speech the consonants are of higher pitch than the vowels. The patient may interpret a word like 'pear' as though it were 'bear' to give one example. This can seem funny to the observer but not to the deaf person who believes that other people think he is stupid. Then people begin to shout at him, which does not he in the least, as he still cannot make out the consonants and he is embarrassed by the attention drawn to him. After a while the deaf person stops trying to communicate and becomes silent and withdrawn. As his deafness worsens he may become depressed or paranoid. He sits watching other people talking, laughing and looking towards him and he becomes convinced that they are talking about him. Brooding enlarges his delusions and his silent world may become peopled with fantasies that everyone is against him. This is an extreme case, and many deaf people bear their affliction good naturedly, but deafness probably is responsible for more misery than any other defect.

What can the Nurse do to Help?

What can the nurse do to help? The first thing is to observe that the patient is deaf, something which few patients volunteer. Having established the fact the nurse should speak slowly, distinctly and in complete sentences, always facing the patient. One should never shout but if the patient cannot hear ordinary conversation one should speak close to his better ear but still in a normal voice. It is helpful to think of the patient as though he was abroad with only a smattering of the foreign language. He can understand only when the natives speak slowly and distinctly. He does not have to catch every sound as long as he gets the general drift and he can obtain help from watching facial expression and the movements of the lips. One can also communicate by writing.

Deaf patients can sometimes be helped by operations and other special forms of treatment, and may well benefit from a hearing aid. Unfortunately some old people refuse to wear hearing aids because they consider them to be conspicuous and think that they draw attention to their handicap, which is what they want to avoid. Of course this is very foolish of them — it is not their fault that they are deaf but unfortunately people are not always logical. Others use hearing aids for a time but dislike them because they distort the sound of the outside world. The younger patient gets used to this noise and soon fails to notice it but the older person may give up his aid because of it.

Other patients complain of a buzzing sound or of the noise of clothes rubbing against the microphone. Others have difficulty in keeping the ear mould in place and many old patients forget to turn the instrument off when it is not in use, or turn it up too high. This causes it to emit a high pitched whine. Others again, fail to replace their batteries. Patients should be encouraged to persevere until their difficulties are overcome. Many a deaf patient's life can be transformed by the proper use of a hearing aid.

Blindness

At any age blindness is a dreadful handicap. It is particularly poignant when it attacks persons of advanced years depriving them of freedom to get about in the outside world and taking from them the pleasures of reading and watching television. Two common causes of failing sight in old age — cataract and glaucoma — both can be benefited by treatment yet many old people are reluctant to have treatment and need encouragement and persuasion.

Unfortunately many old people have great difficulty in adapting to blindness. It is extremely difficult for them to master Braille which requires very sensitive finger tips and an alert active brain. A simpler form of embossed reading symbols called 'moon type' has been evolved for their use and the more alert should be encouraged to learn this. Blind people can be taught the safest and most practical ways of dressing themselves, feeding, using their kitchen and walking. They can be given special watches, sets of draughts, chess, dominoes and playing cards, even typewriters, which enable them to participate on a level with sighted persons.

They are entitled to certain pension benefits and to the provision of radio sets and other amenities which are obtained through the local Blind Welfare organization.

A recent boon to blind people has been the Talking Book Organisation. The more recent ones incorporate small cassettes.

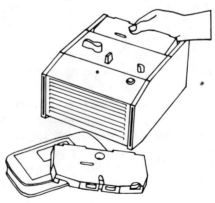

These cassettes contain two tape spools. No threading of the tape is needed making the cassette simple for the blind person to use.

Earphones can be used thus enabling the patient to enjoy a private world of literature, music or language without feeling that the sound may be affecting others.

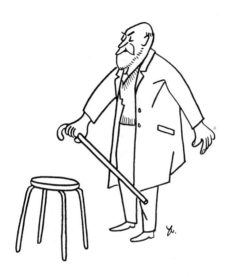

The illustration shows the right way for a blind person to walk, boldly and confidently with the stick held well in front and diagonally along the width of the body so that it will encounter any obstacle before the blind person reaches it.

The Patient's Clothes, Food, etc. Clothes are to be taken off and draped round a chair systematically so that they are there in the same place when next required. Food is to be laid on the plate in the same way with, for example meat on one side and potatoes on the other. Planning, foresight and alertness solve many of the blind patient's problems. But physical illness and mental apathy, when combined with loss of vision, create isolation and despondency.

Dysarthria

In the geriatric ward the nurse will encounter patients who, as a result of a disease affecting the brain, such as a stroke, have lost the power of speech either partially or completely. In one group of cases the speech is merely very indistinct but there is no disturbance of the actual words which the patient is trying to say. This condition is called dysarthria. In some cases the speech sounds like that of a drunken man; in others for example in Parkinson's disease, the voice is very weak and feeble and the words run into one another. Speech therapy can help these cases, and patients can speak better if they are encouraged to take plenty of time. The busy nurse who is addressed by a dysarthric patient and who fails to understand him even after repetition is tempted to say 'yes' and to move on; but will not do so if she thinks of the effect of this on the patient. He becomes disheartened and his attempts to communicate no lapse into the same state of withdrawal as the deaf patient.

Dysphasia and Aphasia

The other type of speech disturbance is much more difficult to understand. In this condition the patient may lose the ability to speak, or the ability to understand speech, or both. The condition may be partial when it is called 'dysphasia' or complete when it is called 'aphasia'. The totally aphasic patient can neither speak or understand what is said to him. Usually he cannot read or write either and sometimes he cannot even understand gestures or situations around him. Other aphasic patients understand at least some of what is said and may be very cleve at picking up clues. Their hearing is not often affected and nurses shoul never shout at them or talk about them in their presence. Some understand everything that is said. Aphasic patients may be able to say only a few words — sometimes the same word over and over again. Some say 'yes' in answer to every question, others similarly say 'no' and it is easy to misinterpret their meaning. Others have quite a free flow of speech but the words are all jumbled up and make little sense. Patients who know what they want to say but who are unable to get the right words out can become very frustrated and exasperated. *Most nurses learn to be skilful at interpreting the wishes of the aphasic patient,* but their ss of language skill cuts them off from the enjoyment of so much of ormal living that they go through phases of deep depression. It is xtremely important for the nurse to treat the aphasic patient with xceptional thoughtfulness, so as to make him believe that his handicap as not completely cut him off from the companionship of his fellow- en.

The few who can read and write should be given every opportunity o do so.

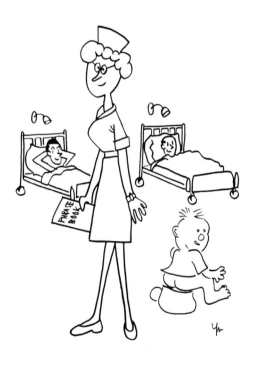

Most nurses learn to be skilful at interpreting the wishes of the aphasic patient — old or young.

Intellectual Deprivation

This is all too common in geriatric patients. As the years go by their brains become less active, their memories fade, they lose their awarene of what is happening among them and they finally become apathetic and isolated. But it is astonishing how much of this can be recovered b stimulating the patient. A ward party, a hair-do, a new dress, a bus outing, a sing-song can transform these patients at least temporarily an can greatly improve their power of communication.

Physical Difficulties

These also deprive many handicapped patients of the opportunity to communicate. The non-ambulant patient can only talk to those who come to him and if he is left alone, either at home or in a hospital day room, he has nothing to say and no one to say it to. Mobilization transforms him as a personality, giving him things to talk about and companionship. Mere transfer from an upstairs house to a ground floor one likewise can remove many problems of communication.

Confidential Information

Finally the nurse should be concerned that the patient communicates those matters which are of concern to him. Patients have many fears and anxieties about their health, their homes, their money, their loved ones, but may be shy to talk of such matters to doctors, even the medical social worker. So they talk instead of symptoms. They may say 'I have a headache' when they really mean 'I am worried about my daughter'. The act of communication is to penetrate into the recesses o the patient's mind and read his secret doubts and fears. This is the nurse's opportunity and her privilege.

She must guard and protect the confidences which she is given and disclose them only to those she can trust if she feels that to do this will help the patient's long term well being.

Diet and Feeding

Old people's bodies are made out of the food they eat. If they eat unwisely their bodies will suffer. Many old people do eat wrongly. A basic knowledge of dietary principles can help nurses to give better care to their elderly patients.

Principles of Dietetics

From the point of view of dietetics food consists of three main elements — protein, carbohydrates and fat.

Protein

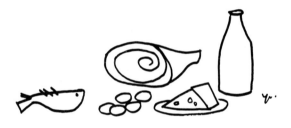

The basic material of living matter — protein — is found in meat, fish, eggs, milk, cheese and certain cereals and vegetables. The body uses protein for growth and repair of its tissues. It is possible for an old person to live without protein or with only a very small amount for a considerable time, but a diet which fails to provide adequate protein leads to a general deterioration of health and to wasting of the muscles.

Carbohydrates

These provide the body with its main source of energy. Carbohydrate foods are also known as sugars and starches and they include sugar itself, sweets, chocolates, cakes, biscuits, bread, rice, cereals, preserves, pastries.

Root vegetables, such as potatoes, also contain a lot of carbohydrate. A lack of carbohydrate in the diet does no real harm at all but the person who takes insufficient carbohydrate will most probably be eating a diet that fails to meet his energy requirements, so he will feel hungry and listless and will lose weight. It is more common for people to eat too much carbohydrate. This is what causes obesity.

Fat

This does not mean only the visible fat such as that which is present in meat, but also the fat in fish, nuts, milk etc. This category also includes butter, margarine, cooking fats and vegetable oils. These *fats* do not necessarily make people fat. It is rather an excess of carbohydrates in the diet that is responsible for obesity. Dietary fat, especially fat of vegetable origin is essential for the maintenance of health.

Minerals and Vitamins

In addition to these three main ingredients, a healthy diet must contain adequate amounts of minerals and vitamins.

Minerals

Minerals are chemical substances used in building body tissues. The two most important from the point of view of the diet of old people are *iron* and *calcium.*

Iron

This is the mineral that the body uses to form blood. It is present especially in meat, eggs, vegetables and oatmeal. If there is insufficient in the diet the patient becomes anaemic; this type is called iron-deficient anaemia. Iron is especially necessary for people who are losing blood, e.g. during the child bearing years, people with bleeding piles, even people taking aspirins regularly who may lose small unnoticed amounts of blood from the gastro-intestinal tract.

Calcium

Calcium is used for building bones and teeth. It is contained in dairy

roduce and flour. If the diet lacks calcium or if too much calcium is
st from the body as occurs in some diseases e.g. after stomach opera-
ons, then the bones may soften. This is a common cause of back pain.

Vitamins

hese are chemical substances required by the body in tiny amounts, so
ttle that one never sees a vitamin; yet without them some important
hemical process in the body cannot take place and diseases result.

Vitamins A and the vitamins of Group B are present in adequate
mount in most diets.

Vitamin C, which maintains general health and keeps the walls of the
lood vessels in good condition is present mainly in milk, fruit,
otatoes, and fresh vegetables. Vitamin C is destroyed by prolonged
ooking. The diet of old people is often deficient in this vitamin.

Vitamin D is required for the maintenance of strong bones. It is
resent in variable amounts in fats such as butter but is added in con-
tant amount to margarine.

Lack of Vitamin D is a common cause of disease in the aged.

To give some idea of the relative amounts that are needed of various
ood elements, old people require about 150G of carbohydrate a day,
0G of protein, one-thousandth of a gramme of iron and one-hundred-
housandth of a gramme of vitamin B12.

Milk

Milk is an allround food — in that it contains some of each of these
equirements for a balanced diet.

Calories

Calories are a measure of how much energy or fuel any given amounts
f food provide. For example one gramme of carbohydrate provides four
alories, one slice of bread yields 50 calories. An old person's daily diet
hould give about one thousand five hundred calories. If the diet
rovides an excess of calories, then the food which cannot be burned up
n the body is converted into fat and stored, causing obesity. If the diet
rovides insufficient calories the energy required is obtained by using
tored fat and weight is lost.

Finally all foods contain material which the body cannot digest or absorb and which therefore must be excreted in the stools. This is called roughage and it consists mainly of fibres and cellulose which are present in fruit, vegetables and cereals. This gives bowel motions their 'bulk'.

Dietary Habits

Dietary habits, which may not necessarily have been ideal in earlier life change with altered circumstances, in advanced years.

Old people have less money to spend on food, less energy to enjoy shopping and cooking, and often just cannot be bothered to prepare adequate meals.

Additional adverse factors are poor or absent teeth, loneliness, apathy, food fads, fear of constipation, and depression.

For example a widowed woman often feels that it is not worth whil cooking for one. As she takes less to eat so she becomes under-nourish and easily tired.

Fluid Intake

Ill old people also need a good fluid intake, because in some cases the kidney is less efficient than it is in younger patients and the body is not so good at conserving its necessary fluids. Some old people fail to drink enough for their needs because they do not experience thirst when they are short of fluid; and some are reluctant to drink because they do not wish to have to use the toilet frequently. Old people must have between one and two litres of fluid daily (it matters little in what form). In hot weather they need two litres to make up for the loss in sweat.

Dietary Needs of Old People

The dietary needs of the elderly can be met by following these simple rules.

1 Eat three proper meals a day, of which at least two contain meat, fish, eggs or cheese
2 Do not eat between meals, but drink at any time

3 Drink at least one half pint of milk daily
4 Use margarine instead of butter
5 Eat fresh fruit, salads and vegetables
6 Eat potatoes lightly boiled or steamed
7 Watch your weight

The nurse should try to find out what patients actually eat at home, and part of rehabilitation should be to advise on shopping, cooking and eating habits. She should report on the patient's teeth, observe what is eaten and what is left on the plate, and try to meet the patient's likes without reducing the nutritional value of the diet. A supply of water or fruit juice should always be available both at the bedside and in the day room, and milky drinks should be offered as well as or instead of tea at mid-morning, mid-afternoon and in the evenings. Patients should be encouraged to eat fresh fruit.

Feeding

The routine of patient's meals depends on the circumstances of each hospital but it is best for the patient to move to a separate dining area, visiting the bathroom en route. *The food is served attractively* as it would be in the patient's own home and choice is offered whenever possible.

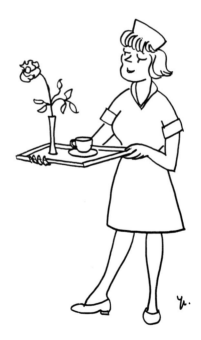

Protection of Clothing

As discreetly as possible the patient's clothing should be protected.

A paper napkin may be enough for some patients but others will require some type of bib or feeder. There are many varieties of these available. The adult 'Pelican Bib' in strong polythene fastening securely at the back of the neck catches drips and food particles very adequately but is very much resented by some patients, nevertheless. other patients e.g. a hemiplegic patient will be glad to use it, secure in the knowledge that his clothing will not be spoiled.

Plastic 'Dental Bibs' are useful as they have a turn-up at the bottom There are also disposable paper bibs with a light plastic backing.

Complaints

Complaints should be listened to patiently — they are often reasonable and can be rectified. Encouragement and help should be given to slow and reluctant feeders, and note should be taken of those who eat poorly — this is a valuable indication of their general health.

Smoking

Most hospitals adopt a permissive attitude to smoking after meals. Ash trays should be provided.

Bed Patients

Bed patients should be positioned comfortably so that they can reach the food on their tray easily. A proportion of patients require to be fe and relatives may help in this time consuming task.

Aids to Feeding

For the nurse the best aid to feeding is a liquidiser as some of her patients may well be on semi-solid diet.

For the patient there are many gadgets on the market to assist feeding. Most patients hate to appear conspicious, moreover there is always the problem of gadgets being lost when they are washed up, so it is better to avoid their use whenever possible. The following have been found valuable.

Non-slip Mats
These are made of a 'tacky' plastic or a polyurethane web. They prevent the plate from slipping while the patient with only one effective hand chases an elusive piece of meat around the plate.

Bowls
For patients who are liable to spill their food over the edge of the plate, a deep bowl is preferred to a clip-on 'plate bunker'.

Spork
This is a combined spoon and fork. Similar inventions for the one-handed patient include the combined knife and fork.

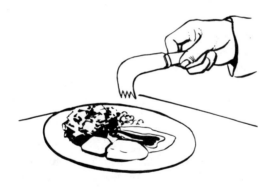

The Flexible Straw
This is used by patients with severe tremor (eg in Parkinson's disease) who are unable to hold a cup.

Many firms these days are doing a great deal of research into these things and the nurse would be advised to check from time to time in manufacturer's publications for the latest developments.

Diets

Most patients are on a normal mixed diet.

Patients on a special diet should be listed; and in order to minimize errors they should be advised themselves of what they may and may no eat. In some hospitals, individual diets are sent up from the diet kitchen in others the ward staff must make up the diet with the guidance of a diet sheet. This may be one of several forms:

1 An *exact* diet giving the precise food and the quantities to be served
2 A diet similar to (1) but with alternative foods and quantities.
3 A list of permitted and prohibited foods, with quantities not exactly specified.

The diets commonly used are:

1 Diabetic Diet
2 High Protein Diet
3 Low Protein Diet
4 High Residue Diet
5 Low Fat Diet
6 Low Salt Diet
7 High Calcium Diet
8 Reduction Diet

Diabetic Diet

The restriction of calorie intake and in particular carbohydrate — is dependent on the degree of severity of the diabetes.

Some cases can be controlled this way. Others require diet in addition to drug therapy.

High Protein Diet

This contains extra meat, fish, eggs, milk and cheese. It is used for malnourished patients, and also for weight reduction. Special protein supplements can be added.

Low Protein Diet

This diet is used for patients with kidney and liver diseases. Since cereal foods and bread contain a significant amount of protein, the choice of foods is very narrow and rice and fruit are the main constituents.

High Residue Diet

This is advocated for the prevention of constipation, and for the treatment of disorders of the large bowel. The diet contains wholemeal bread, raw fruit and vegetable, All Bran and Weetabix.

Low Fat Diet

This is prescribed for patients with disease of the gall bladder and in some cases of liver disease. Because of the reduction in butter and cooking fat it is difficult to make a palatable diet.

Low Salt Diet

This is prescribed in some cases of heart disease and high blood pressure. Little salt is used in cooking, none may be added at the table.

High Calcium Diet

This is used to treat some bone diseases. Extra milk and cheese are given.

Reduction Diet

In this the total number of calories is given eg a reduction diet which provides 1000 calories or less — some as little as 400 calories. In a diabetic diet the total amount of carbohydrate only is sometimes fixed, eg 100 grammes and in others the protein and fat content are also laid down and guidance is given on the diet sheet.

8
Clothing and Personal Care

Every nurse knows personally the boost to morale which comes from being smartly dressed. Ill old people feel just as good as anyone else when they are well turned out, especially when they have just put their clothes on for themselves and appreciate a compliment. Geriatric wards require and usually have adequate wardrobe space. Relatives should be advised on the best kind of clothes to bring in and told to label them clearly and to be responsible for alterations and repairs.

It is a part of the patient's treatment that he should learn to dress himself and only those patients should be dressed by the nurses who are designated as requiring this help. When patients return home relatives are only too prone to dress them, unless the patient's will to do this for himself has been strongly trained in hospital.

Dresses and suits especially
designed for incontinent and
disabled patients are now
available:

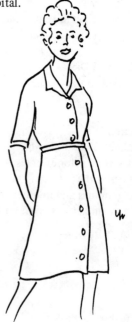

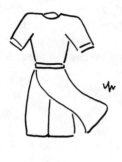

The skirts have overlaps, or back panels and the fastenings are simple and easily reached, eg cross-over skirts and button through dresses.

All these garments are made from easy-care fabrics which are available in a large range of colours and patterns.

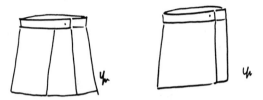

Crimplene and terylene trousers are available for men.

Dressing Difficulties

These may be due to one or a combination of the following:

Loss of movement of one or more limbs as a result of hemiplegia etc.

Loss of range of movement at joints as a result of arthritis, bone injury etc.

Loss of perception as a result of blindness or in some cases of stroke where for example, the patient loses the ability to identify the different parts of his garments and to relate them to the parts of his body.

Loss of balance, as a result of stroke, Parkinson's disease, etc. when the patient cannot sit unsupported, stand on one leg or reach far forward — all movements which are used in normal dressing.

Loss of strength, as in heart and chest diseases, when the patient becomes exhausted by the physical effort of dressing.

Loss of memory as in cases of brain disease, such as stroke and dementia, when the patient does not remember the sequence of movements necessary to put a garment on, and may waste his efforts in a disconnected series of ineffective movements.

Loss of awareness also found in some cases of stroke and dementia, where the patient puts his clothes on in an absurd manner, eg back to front or in the wrong order.

Loss of will to help oneself, as in depression, when the patient makes no attempt to dress or insists that he cannot. The nurse should therefore watch the patient struggling with his clothes and make up her mind, using the knowledge of his illness to help her, to decide which of the above is the cause of his inability to dress. Once this is known ways can be found to help.

However, detailed dressing training in a difficult case is a matter for the occupational therapist.

It is desirable for an older person to have a chair with arms but in the interests of clarity in the illustration chair arms are left out.

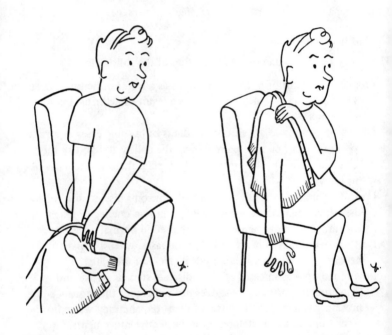

Patients with weakness of one upper limb or with limitation of movement of one shoulder joint are taught to put the bad arm into its sleeve first, then to pull the garment over the head or round the back with the good hand and finally to put the good arm through its sleeve.

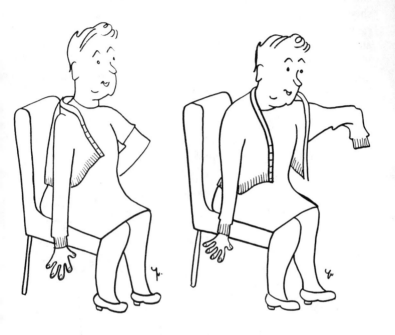

The hand of the bad arm is then laid on the lap.
In undressing the good arm is taken out first, the bad arm last.

Patients with visual difficulties can be helped by sewing on a large white patch to indicate the part that is to be put on first, eg the lining of the arm hole of a jacket.

Patients with balance difficulties can dress while lying on top of their beds. Those who easily become exhausted should dress partially and the nurse should help them before they become tired or breathless.

Garments should be few, warm and simple. Some may need to be specially adapted. The clothes should be laid out in the order in which they are to be worn.

Men should wear vest, shorts, sports shirt, pullover or cardigan, slacks, socks, slip on shoes; but as they improve they may introduce shirts with buttons, collar and tie, trousers with braces, jacket, lacing shoes.

Women should use vest and pants, slip, button front dress or jumper and skirt or slacks if preferred. Tights or grip top stockings should be worn. Low heeled lacing shoes (with elastic laces) are required. As they improve they can introduce brassieres and other under garments, girdles, suspenders and different styles of frock.

Detachable Suspender

The suspender is attached to the stocking, and after the stocking has been put on, the suspender is hooked on to the girdle.

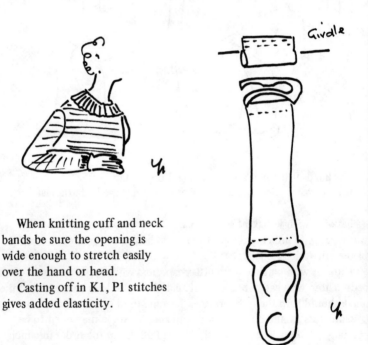

When knitting cuff and neck bands be sure the opening is wide enough to stretch easily over the hand or head.

Casting off in K1, P1 stitches gives added elasticity.

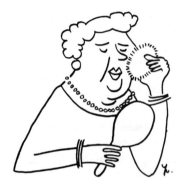

Nothing is better for a patient's
morale than to feel well groomed
and well dressed.

Laundering Arrangements

The value of the patient wearing his own clothes and thus boosting his morale has already been mentioned.

It is the identification of each person's clothes which raises problems for the nursing staff. The clothing of each patient should be clearly labelled with his name, the ward number and, if the clothing goes to a group laundry, the name of the hospital.

Each patient should have an individual locker or wardrobe for his clothes.

Relatives should be encouraged to take clothes home for washing but if this is not possible the clothing must be washed at the hospital laundry.

Skirts, woollens and trousers — unless specifically shown as washable — should be dry cleaned.

Nowadays the increasing range of drip-dry washable garments is especially useful for the incontinent patient.

Few hospital laundries are equipped to deal with drip-dry materials and in many cases these things are washed at ward level.

Some Geriatric Units have their own washing machine or spin/ tumbler dryer.

Fastenings

Fastenings provide difficulty for weak and stiff fingers.

Zips and hooks and eyes are particularly awkward, especially for patients who do not have full use of both hands. They should be replaced by large buttons or by strips of Velcro. A brassiere which normally fastens at the back by awkward hooks and eyes can be converted into one which fastens easily in front by Velcro.

What is Velcro?

Velcro touch and close fastener consists of two nylon strips, one a mass of tiny hooks and the other a mass of tiny loops. When placed together the hooks grip the loops to give a tight, secure closure — yet the two strips can easily be separated by pulling them apart.

It is available in a variety of colours and in different widths. It may be used as a straight-forward fastener, in strips or small pieces, as an alternative to buttons, which is far easier to open and close as they do not require such precise positioning.

Velcro has value in allowing garments to be adjusted for size, or to provide additional unobtrusive openings where these ease dressing.

Like tape, Velcro may be hand or machine sewn to fabric, or even 'glued on' with a contact adhesive. The loop side is softer than the hook side and should be the one facing the skin, although it is advisable to ensure that this fastening does not have contact with the skin in the usual way, as it is abrasive by its nature.

Washing of Velcro is quite straight-forward and requires no special measures except closure of the fastening before it is washed. If this is not done Velcro picks up fluff and the hooks and loops become clogged, when the fastener ceases to work properly. It may be washed or dry-cleaned.

Extreme pressure will damage Velcro.

Ironing should be with a warm iron.

Velcro applied with clear adhesive will stand up to home laundering.

Velcro is not always satisfactory in use on woollen garments as it tends to adhere to the garment. When Velcro adheres to woollen fabric it becomes clogged with fluff.

Velcro peels open easily.

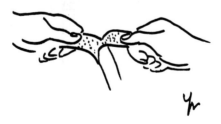

Velcro grips firmly giving a secure closure of the garment.

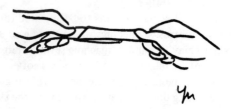

Wrap-around skirt either back or front fastening fastened with pieces of Velcro.

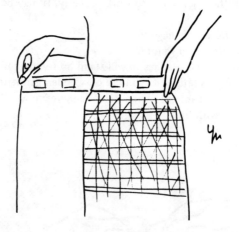

Velcro used with belt and buckle fastening.

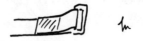

Front fastening of brassiere using Velcro.

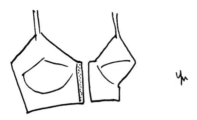

This garment is fastened at the back with strips of Velcro.

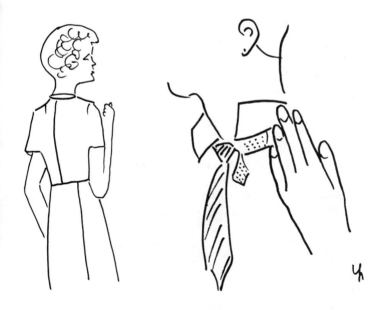

Velcro can be used for an easy tie fastening.

Zips

Zips can be difficult to manage and should be placed as conveniently as possible.

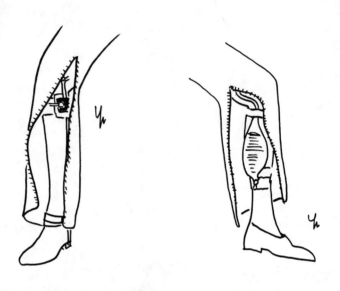

The illustration shows the outer seam of a trouser leg incorporating a zip fastener. This greatly helps the patient who wears calipers.

A zip fastener side-opening is a great help to the wearer of incontinence apparatus.

Zip fasteners obviously make excellent substitutes for the fly in trousers.

Open Ended Zip

A zip fastener with an openable end means that many garments which might otherwise need to go over the head can be put on in a jacket-like fashion.

This is a good method of helping someone to manage their own zip at the back of a dress.

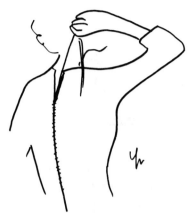

A piece of cord or firm tape is passed through the metal loop of the slider cap.

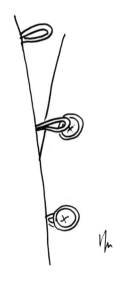

Buttons

Buttons can be sewn on using elastic thread. This makes them easier for disabled patients to fasten.

Loop buttonholes made either from cord, material or firm elastic are easier than bound buttonholes.

Toggle Buttons

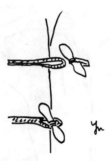

These are easy to handle. The loop is made from cord and the toggles are usually made in natural wood.

Velcro 'Buttons'

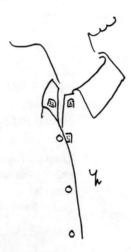

Any buttoned garment can be adapted as shown to pieces of Velcro thus keeping the appearances normal.

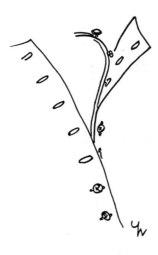

Sew the button on a tape and with an extra row of buttonholes where the buttons would normally be sewn — the operation of the removal of the buttons on the tape is easy.

Expanding Cuff Links

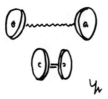

These can be made from two buttons and threaded with fine tubular elastic. They can then be left in position in the cuff of the shirt when it is put on and taken off.

Hooks

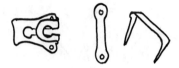

The bar and hook can only be used in firm or backed materials. There is no sewing involved as the bar points are pressed through the material and the locking bar attached and the points of the bar are then folded down.

The hook is of course sewn on to the garment.

Shoe Fastening

This can be a most serious difficulty to the frail or hemiplegic patient.

The following illustrations show simply how shoes can be firmly laced using one hand.

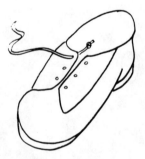

Knot the end of a leather lace.

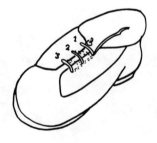

Thread slackly.
To tighten pull 2, 3, and end.

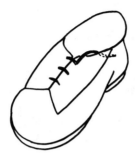

Tuck end of lace down inside of shoe.

Elastic Shoe Laces
The need for these has largely disappeared with the wide availability of slip on shoes.

Long Handled Shoe Horn

A long handled shoe horn with flexible tubing between handle and shoe horn, to assist patient who has only one useful hand or who has difficulty in bending.

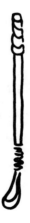

Elastic Waist Bands

Elastic is often used as alternative fastenings.

Special elastic edges for trousers, underpants, or knickers.

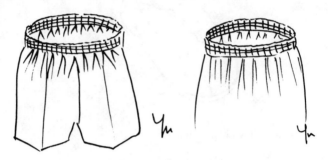

A skirt made from tweed with an elasticised edge.

Clip-on Apron

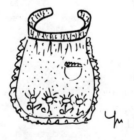

It is very difficult to tie an apron at the back and even quite difficult to fix the ends with Velcro so a clip-on apron has become a great boon to handicapped people.

Gadgets

Many gadgets have been devised to assist in dressing. The following are the most useful:

Stocking Aids

These are of various types — the simpler the better. Their value is limited because the patient may find it difficult to attach the stocking to the aid. They are of special help to patients with arthritis and with balance disturbances who cannot possibly lean forward.

Dressing Stick

This is simply a stick with a padded end (a padded coat hanger is satisfactory) which can help a patient with a weak or stiff arm to struggle with awkward sleeves.

Made-up Ties

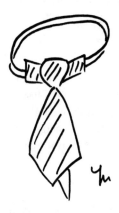

These can either be of the type shown or of a made-up tie mounted on elastic which will hold it snugly under the collar.

Gadgets can be helpful but are easily lost, mislaid or broken and the aim should be to reserve them for the patients who cannot dress without them.

Washing Difficulties

Washing poses difficulties similar to those described under dressing. The main problems encountered are those due to loss of power in one hand or arm, limitation of shoulder movements, disturbance of balance, and dementia.

Useful Gadgets
1 Magnetic soap holder
2 Glove sponge
3 Long-handled sponge
4 Long-handled loofah
5 Long-handled back-brush

Towels
Roller towels are easiest for one-handed patients. Alternatively an ordinary towel with tapes sewn on and tied to hooks on the wall serves the purpose.

Bathing Difficulties

Bathing presents many difficulties to the frail old person. Many are afraid to risk taking a bath, and prefer a bed bath or a wash-down. Sitting baths, cabinet baths and showers all have their supporters and their opponents. But since most old people and most nurses in the United Kingdom are used to the conventional plunge bath this will be dealt with first.

Precautions
1 Frail old people should not be left in the bathroom alone.
2 Water temperature should be tested *most carefully* with the hand and with a thermometer. In baths with thermostatically controlled mixing valves the temperature should be set at 38–39°C but it is still desirable to check the actual temperature of the water in the bath.
3 Make sure that the bathroom floor is dry.
4 Patients should never grip the taps to pull themselves up in the bath.
5 All electrical fittings must be carefully checked.

Bathing Routine

1 The patient is prepared for the bath by being undressed and covered with night-gown and blankets.

2 He is brought to the bathroom in a chair or by a lifting apparatus (Ambulift).

3 A rubber non-slip mat is placed on the bottom of the bath.

4 The bath is filled to a suitable depth with water of the correct temperature (38–39°C).

5 The patient enters the bath using one of the methods described below.

6 The patient is supported in the bath and is thoroughly washed.

7 He is covered with a towel while the bath is emptied.

8 Once the water has drained out he leaves the bath by one of the methods to be described.

9 He is thoroughly dried, powdered, dressed and returned to bed

10 The bath is washed down thoroughly with an ordinary domestic cleaning agent.

A hand held shower situated close to the bath can be used for hair washing and for washing patients in the bath — but please regulate the temperature of the water carefully.

Frail patients and heavy ones are bathed more easily with the help of a patient hoist. The following procedure relates to the 'Ambulift' which has proved very useful, but there are several other types of patient-lifting apparatus on the market, many of them considerably cheaper. Nursing staff require a good deal of training and experience before mastering the use of these complex aids; and special time should be made available for this training because in the long run the correct use of lifting apparatus is a great saver of time and strength. It is easier on the patient giving him a sense of security and comfort and on the nurse saving her a great deal of heavy lifting.

What is an Ambulift?

It provides manoeuvrability and transport for almost any patient no matter what the disablement or physical limitation. It can be aptly

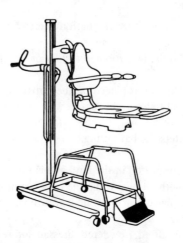

described as a complete patient handling system.

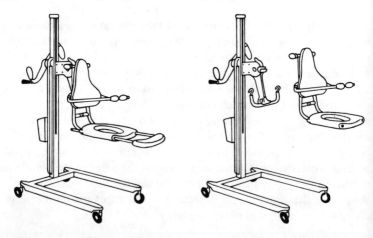

The chair unit has no legs of its own, and is freely detachable from the lift/transporter section. This serves two purposes: firstly, it makes for easier 'loading' and 'unloading' of the patient at the bed, and also without disturbing the patient it makes it possible to convert the seat into a commode, sanitary or shower-bath chair.

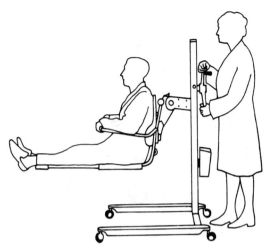

To lift a man is one of the most difficult physical tasks a nurse is called upon to perform. It is also undignified for the patient. Thousands of nurses must have suffered permanent injury themselves, doing this work. This danger has been partly eliminated with the advent of the Ambulift.

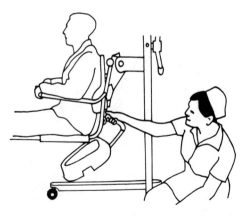

There is a toiletting device which is easy to use and most acceptable to the patients.

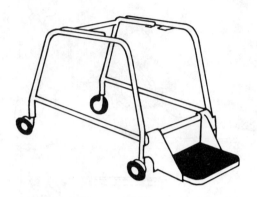

There is a stainless steel sub-chassis which can be used to convert the chair for toilet or shower use.

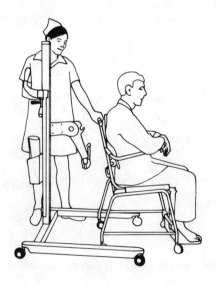

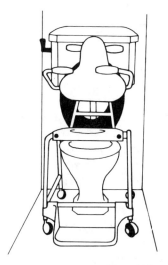

The Patient using an Ambulift as a bathing Aid.

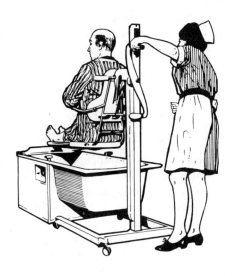

85

Procedure for Bathing with the Ambulift

1 Fill the bath one third full of water at a temperature 38°–39°C
2 Take Ambulift to side of bed
3 Roll patient to opposite side of the bed
4 Lower Ambulift seat to level of the bed and roll patient on to it
5 Sit patient up on seat and place Ambulift arms round patient
6 Wind up seat from bed level and move Ambulift to bathroom positioning seat directly above the end of the bath
7 Remove patient's clothing
8 Lower seat with patient into the bath
9 Move Ambulift arms back and wash patient
10 Replace Ambulift arms and raise seat to above bath
11 Dry the patient
12 Put on clothing
13 Return patient to bed on Ambulift

Procedure for bathing with a Bath Seat

Patients who are able to sit and stand unsupported but who lack the balance and confidence to enter a bath in the normal way require a simple bathing aid consisting of a broad board which lies across the top of the bath and a seat which sits inside the bath. The technique of using this system is as follows.

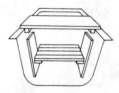

1 The patient is brought to the bathroom in a wheel chair
2 The board is secured across the bath near its top end; the seat is wedged into the bath a little further down
3 The patient transfers (see chapter 4) from the wheelchair to sit on the bath board facing away from the bath. If the bath is not set against the wall so that there is a choice of sides, she enters the bath from her better side. A patient with left hemiplegia enters the left side of the bath.

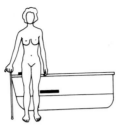

4 She works her bottom back on the board until she is sitting over the middle of the bath

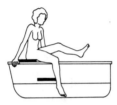

5 She swings her legs up and round into the bath, if necessary tucking the stronger leg under the weaker one

6 Steadying herself with the hand grips she slips on to the seat.

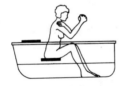

7 She is then bathed while sitting on the seat and she may allow herself to slip right down on to the bottom of the bath. The hand-held shower will help to give her a refreshing bath

8 After she has been bathed the bath is emptied

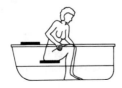

87

9 The patient uses the hand grip to step up from the stool to the board. (If there is no grip then she will lean forward, put hand well back on edge of bath; push straight up and back on to board.)
10 She slides to the right, lifts her right leg out of the bath

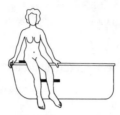

11 Her left leg follows and now she is sitting on the bath board facing out of the bath
12 She is dried and transferred back to the wheel chair

Steadier patients may dispense with the bath board but will welcome the hand grips across the bath, at the side of the bath or on the wall. These can be vertical, horizontal or diagonal according to desire, but should be about 7 cm in diameter to give a good grip, and should preferably be covered with ribbed rubber grip. A mat at the bottom of the bath and a dry floor or carpet are always essential.

Other Bathing Aids for Mobile Patients

Simplex Bath Seat

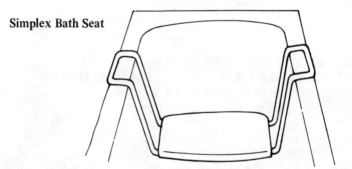

This aid adapts to the bath to help those patients who find difficulty in getting into or out of the bath. Rubber covered rests prevent scratching bath sides.

Economic Bath Seat

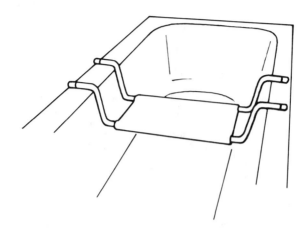

This is made of stout steel tube covered with protective plastic, and tested to carry forty stones with safety.

The OB Karin Bath Seat

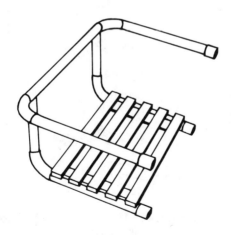

Bath Handle

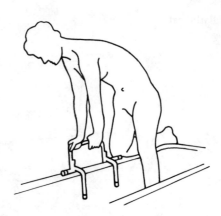

Adjustable Bath Handle

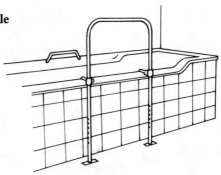

Bath Safety Mat

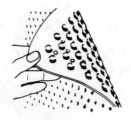

Completely safe and comfortable. Hundreds of small suction cups hold the mat securely to the bottom of the bath.

Sitting Baths

Sitting baths overcome many of the difficulties of the conventional bath.

The Medic Bath

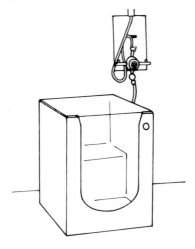

The Medic Bath is essentially a sitting bath with a removable front panel covering the gap through which a patient can enter over a shallow step. This bath is particularly useful for patients who cannot lift their feet easily and is best used with a shower.

The Ladywell Bath System

The Ladywell Bath System is designed for more severely handicapped patients who can be wheeled into the bath in a specially designed chair. The end door is then closed and the bath filled. To make things easier for nurses washing severely handicapped patients, the bath can be installed at the right working height. When nurses have a variety of equipment on each ward they can also experiment using different bits of equipment in combination — the Ambulift hoist with the Ladywell Bath, for instance.

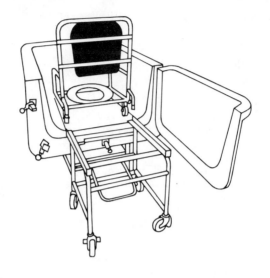

In these the patient enters the bath on a special bathing chair through a door, this is then closed and the bath is filled rapidly. After he has been washed the waste water is pumped out, the door is re-opened and the patient is wheeled out again.

Shower Tables

Some severely handicapped patients find it frightening to be brought to the bath by a hoist, dislike being placed in an empty bath before it is filled, or are too handicapped to use any of the systems already mentioned. Swedish shower table systems could help these patients. One model has an adjustable-height platform which can be taken to the bedside to move the patient to the shower or bathroom. The patient is then showered horizontally on the platform—adjusted to give varying degrees of 'backrest'. After bathing the patient returns to bed on the platform. The platform surfaces are made of plastic material which can be easily brought to body temperature and which dries quickly.

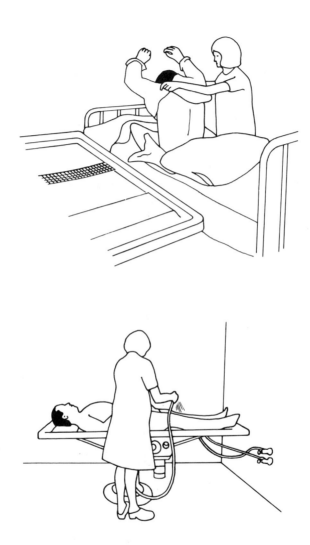

These systems could be most useful for the care of severely handicapped patients.

Showers

Showers have many advantages for bathing. The most convenient form is the *shower room* which has a slightly sloping floor and a drain. The patient is simply brought into the room on a special wheelchair, or transferred on to a shower stool and the attendant showers him using a hand held shower. A shower compartment is less satisfactory, the disadvantage being the presence of a kerb, the slippery porcelain floor and the lack of room for manoeuvre. Few geriatric patients can stand safely in a shower bath even when hand grips are provided, and transferring them safely from a wheel chair to a shower stool in a limited space over a kerb and a slippery floor is not very easy. Moreover many older patients are frightened in a shower; some find it cold; others complain that they do not feel they have had a real bath! and finally the attendant gets very wet unless she is suitably clad.

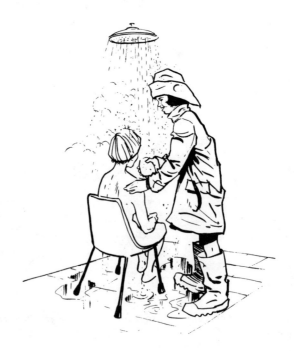

Accurate regulation of water temperature is essential in a shower bath and great care must be taken that the water does not suddenly become hotter because a cold tap has been turned on somewhere else, with a resultant drop in the cold water pressure in the mixture of water in the shower. A thermostatically controlled mixing valve is an essential safety feature.

Soiled Patients

A special problem in geriatric nursing is created by the patient who soils himself while he is up and dressed. He has to be taken to the bathroom and washed and changed. It is obviously undesirable that this cleansing operation should take place in the ordinary bathroom, but it is sometimes not practical to make special provision in existing hospitals although new hospitals will have a cleansing room specially designed for this purpose.

A toilet-bidet type fixture which allows the patient to sit forward and thus permit the nurse to clean him from behind with a hand operated shower is useful in this situation.

There is not at present, nor is there ever likely to be, any wholly satisfactory method of bathing all frail geriatric patients. The best solution is for each unit to have available more than one method, so that patients can be dealt with according to their individual requirements and preferences.

Care of the Hair

Care of the hair is much more than the conventional examination for parasites (or head lice) although regrettably this feature cannot be over-looked and when they are found they should be dealt with by daily combing with a fine tooth comb and the application of Lorexane. It is very important that all nits are removed. Ordinary care of the hair is as necessary for geriatric patients as it is for anyone else in order to give a smart attractive appearance and a sense of pride and dignity. A hair drier is as necessary a piece of equipment in a geriatric ward as a thermometer; and it sometimes appears to doctors that a "hair do" is a more effective way of treating depression in the elderly female than is a course of electric convulsion therapy.

Patients should be encouraged to do their own hair, and there should be an adequate number of mirrors. For the handicapped, especially patients with arthritis of the shoulders, long handled brushes and combs can be invaluable. A weekly shampoo need never be omitted except in the extremely ill.

Care of the Nails
Care of the nails is of similar importance.

The toe nails especially are frequently neglected by ill old people and every nurse will see the condition known as *onychogryphosis* in which the neglected nail overgrows to an enormous extent until it is a great curved shaggy unsightly horn. Nurses can deal with ordinary nail clipping, taking great care to cut the nail straight across and avoiding damage to the skin. They should not attempt to deal with any abnormality such as a corn and they should not cut the nails of diabetic patients or of those with vascular disease. These cases should be referred to the chiropodist because there is a special danger that injury might lead to infection and gangrene.

Care of the Teeth
Patients require encouragement in the use of the tooth brush.

Dentures can be labelled by rubbing a part of the plate with emery paper, writing the patients name on it with a ball point pen and applying a coating of nail varnish.

At night the denture is kept in a labelled receptacle at the bedside immersed in a cleaning fluid, such as 'Milton' or 'Steradent', which should be made up with cold water.

9
Sleep and Wakefulness

When we consider the disturbances to which geriatric patients are subjected, it is surprising that any of them ever sleep at all. Here they are, taken away from home and familiar surroundings, many of them in pain or breathless, lying in a strange bed. All around them are snores, sighs and shouts of the other patients, the movement of screens or commodes; the noise of lifts or trolleys from outside the wards, the dim lights and the strange shadows. During the day they have had very little fresh air or exercise and may have spent part of the time dozing in a chair. Their minds are full of anxiety and fear for their health, their future, their homes and families. Their bladders are filling up and they know that sooner or later they will have to summon nurse for help. Yet somehow, the majority of them sleep soundly.

The quality of sleep enjoyed by the patients depends on the work of the night nurse as she settles her patients down. A quiet word with each one in turn helps to give comfort and allays anxiety. One needs an extra pillow, one wants a urinal at the side of the bed, one likes to have cot sides up so that he knows he cannot fall out of bed, another wants his down because they make him feel caged. One must have a drink to settle him, another refuses a drink in case he should need the toilet. One is worried about something the doctor said in the ward round, another because his bowels have not moved. Yet another cannot sleep until he gets his 'pill'. This may be a hypnotic or it may be just an inactive drug, but he won't sleep until he gets it.

After all these individual patients are attended to the night nurse must be free to concentrate on the 'high risk' cases. These are ill and immobile patients; those who are liable to incontinence and those who are subject to confusion and restlessness.

Frequent turning is essential for immobile patients and for them only. The ordinary active person changes his own position in bed frequently even while he is asleep, and then no part of his body is exposed to constant pressure. But ill immobile patients are unable to do this and the weight of their body is transmitted through the pressure points. Unless the patient's position is altered the blood supply at these points of pressure is cut off and *necrosis* of tissue results. This is how pressure sores are caused and the consequences can be disastrous. The patients who need frequent turning are usually ill, heavy and unable to help themselves, and two people will be needed to turn them, ideally every two hours. Night nurses must plan their work carefully and they must waste no time turning people who do not need this. The list of patients requiring two-hourly turning should be reviewed daily.

Prevention and management of incontinence requires just as much vigilance. A wet bed means work for the night nurse. The problem is to find time to wake and commode those patients who are at risk of being incontinent. She should have a list of these patients and she should set aside at least one and preferably two periods in the night for preventive commoding. Patients who are persistently incontinent and who have or are at risk of developing skin troubles are sometimes catheterized.

Two of the most difficult situations with which the night nurse has to deal are the noisy patient and the restless one. Patients who shout all night, who rattle the cot sides, who try to climb out of bed can absorb all the night nurse's attention. Such cases should be reported to the doctor. There may well be a medical cause for the behaviour disturbance such as pneumonia or myocardial infarction. He may be in pain and be unable to express his feelings in any other way. The doctor may recommend treatment which relieves the underlying cause of the patient's condition; or he may order a sedative to control the outburst; or he may arrange for the patient to be removed from the ward altogether.

It is sometimes possible for the night nurse to prevent these noisy outbursts. Some of the noisiest patients have been in the habit of drinking a lot of alcohol and they may settle well with a glass of whisky. In general a sleeping tablet works best if given early in the night at the same time as the patient is settled comfortably in bed. Similarly if a patient has fallen asleep after a hypnotic but then wakes in the middle of the night and becomes noisy, the sooner that further medication is given the more effective it will be. The worst situation and ne that should be avoided, is when the patient is given very large loses of sedation and tranquillizers which only make him even more noisy and confused. They may have a delayed effect, he sleeps all next day and is wakeful and disturbed again the following night. To avoid this situation some doctors use no drugs for disturbed patients and rely instead on simple measures like cups of tea, bars of chocolate and cigarettes.

The behaviour of disturbed patients may be caused by fear. Often they have vivid and frightening dreams and they cannot distinguish dream from reality. Consequently when they waken they still think that they are in the situation of the dream. To their bewilderment cot sides may mean the bars of a prison, nurses may be warders or torturers; and this is why otherwise inoffensive patients can become so vicious and violent. The nurse should try to remain as cool and quiet as possible, to identify herself to the patient, to try to calm and soothe him, to keep the temperature down. The advice is easier to give than to act on in the middle of a busy ward, but it is still the right advice.

The night nurse's job is an arduous one but it is not, and must not be allowed to become mere drudgery. The night nurse plays just as important a part in the patient's management as does the day nurse. Unfortunately it is not so easy for her voice to be heard.

She receives a report when she comes on duty and gives one when she goes off, but she plays little part in the management decisions that are made about the patients and *has few opportunities* of finding out what is wrong with the patients and how they are progressing, except by reading their case sheets.

A periodic meeting between the night nurse, the ward sister and one of the medical staff would help a lot to bridge the communication gap, might well lead to better prescribing and would convey to the night nurse something that she should not have to be told, namely that her skilful observation and management of the patients during the night makes a valuable contribution to the patient's progress by day.

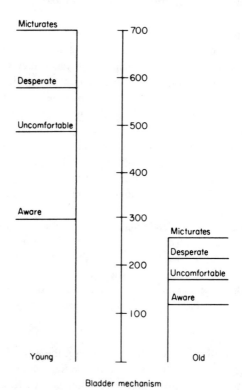

Bladder mechanism

0
The Bladder

The body has complex but efficient mechanisms for ridding itself of its waste products. Unfortunately many diseases which occur in old age impair the efficiency of these mechanisms. A large part of the nursing of geriatric patients is devoted to helping the patient to overcome his difficulties in the evacuation of urine and faeces. The better this part of a nurse's work is done the less time she will have to spend in cleaning up the consequences of failure. This section is therefore concerned primarily with the management of continence and only secondarily with the care of incontinence.

Mechanism of Continence

Why are normal people continent? Because of the way their bladder works. The urinary bladder fills up with urine usually at a rate of between 50 and 150ml an hour by day (depending on fluid intake) and about half this rate by night. Once the volume of urine in the bladder reaches about 300ml the subject becomes aware of urine in the bladder. If he decides not to pass urine the sensation of fullness passes off, but returns again as the bladder capacity increases. By the time the bladder contains 500ml of urine he is definitely uncomfortable, but he can still delay emptying his bladder, despite increasing but intermittent discomfort, until a point is reached when he is, as they say 'desperate'. From then he can manage to hold out a little longer until he has an opportunity of passing urine. When he does he empties his bladder completely.

In geriatric patients many of these mechanisms may be disturbed for a variety of reasons.

1 After micturition the bladder is not fully emptied, but "residual urine" remains in it – commonly there may be 50–100ml. The volume of residual urine depends among other things, on the method of emptying the bladder – it is greater with a bedpan than with a commode or toilet

2 The early sensation of bladder fullness is not perceived

3 The sense of acute discomfort comes on suddenly and without warning

4 The sense of discomfort comes on at small bladder capacity

5 The ability to inhibit the need to pass water is lost

6 The interval between acute discomfort and obligatory emptying of the bladder is very short; in some cases the sensation of acute discomfort is not even perceived

If all these abnormalities are present the patient will suffer from the following symptoms:

1 Frequency – he will pass urine every hour or two instead of every three or four hours
2 Urgency – when he asks for the toilet he will be unable to wait for more than a very short time.
3 Incontinence – he may be unable to prevent his urine passing by itself, or he may be aware of the need to pass urine but have insufficient time to reach the toilet

Some geriatric patients have normal bladder function; and others have different kinds of faults in their bladder-emptying mechanism.

Many are sorely anxious about their bladder and afraid of wetting themselves and of troubling the nurses and this anxiety alone can be responsible for much bladder trouble.

What then can the nurse do to help her patients with bladder troubles?

1 *Allay anxiety*

In many patients the bladder is the biggest worry from the moment when they enter hospital. As soon as they are admitted they should be taken to the toilet, shown exactly where it is in relation to their bed and, if they are fit to do so, they should be told to go as often as they wish. If they are confined to bed or chair they should be advised what to do when they want to use the toilet. They should not wait until they can wait no longer, but should call a nurse the moment they feel the need. They should be told the times of the routine toilet rounds and advised that they will be helped at other times as well. They should be reassured that no one will blame them for any accident. It is not their fault and the nurses do not mind cleaning up. These reassurances must reflect the policy and practice of the nursing staff. Two things which nurses should not say to patients are:

(when asked for a bedpan) — 'I'm too busy now, I'll bring you one later'
(when presented with a wet bed) — 'Why did you wet the bed?'

2 *Ensure Complete Emptying*

A half-empty bladder is a half-full bladder and will need to be emptied again very soon. There are medical causes for incomplete emptying, but some cases are also due to cold, fear, embarrassment or faulty position when passing urine. These are avoided by giving the patient privacy and by using a commode or the toilet in preference to a bedpan.

3 *Ensure Good Communication*

The patient has only a short interval between feeling the need to use the toilet and being unable to avoid wetting himself. If he can walk, seat him near the toilet so that he gets there quickly. If he is in bed be sure that he knows how to use the bell push system and that the bell is close to hand. If he is in the day room do not leave him for more than a short time.

4 Give Prompt Attention

If patients in a day room see one of their members being taken to the toilet they all want to go. The good nurse knows whose request is genuine and who is 'having her on'. If she doesn't she must give the patient the benefit of the doubt.

5 Preventative Toiletting

Make regular toilet rounds every two hours for those in greatest need. I is a lot of work but it saves work in the long run.

6 Keep Patients Physically, Mentally and Socially Fit

The most valuable preventative measure is the general atmosphere of th ward. When the ward is bright and cheerful, the patients are receiving adequate medical attention and rehabilitation, they are smartly dressed in their own clothes, regularly visited and given things to do to occupy themselves, incontinence drops. On the other hand incontinence flourishes in an atmosphere of drabness and despair.

7 Medical Measures

The symptoms of frequency, urgency and incontinence can sometimes be improved or cured by medical and surgical treatment. In the selectio of suitable cases for treatment the doctor needs the best information that nurses can make available to him.

8 An Incontinence Chart

This is a helpful aid to the control of incontinence. Nurses record every time that the patient passes urine whether he was continent or incon- tinent. It is then possible to see at a glance when the incontinence is occurring and what it might be caused by. For example charting in one ward revealed that several patients were being incontinent at about 4 pm on Wednesdays. At that time Wednesday afternoon was the main mid-week visiting period. Patients who needed the toilet did not like to ask while they had visitors. When the visitors left at 4 pm all the patients wanted help at once and those who could not wait were incontinent. In another case the patient was shown by the chart to be always wet at 8 am. He was being wakened at 6 am when he was given a urinal and a cup of tea. After this he fell back into a deep sleep and wet himself while sleeping. Changes in the ward routine solved both these problems.

CONTINENCE CHART

Instructions: Make an entry in the chart each time the patient passes urine, has a
bowel movement or is incontinent by recording the code letters in
the space for that day and hour.

PU—Passes Urine (normally)
PF—Passes faeces (normally)
BW—Bed wet

CW—Clothes wet
BS—Bed soiled (faeces)

CS—Clothes soiled (faeces)
US—Urine spilled
FS—Floor soiled

Name: Ward: Week Commencing:

Time	Monday	Tuesday	Wednesday	Thursday	Friday	Saturday	Sunday
8 a.m.							
9							
10							
11							
Mid-day							
1 p.m.							
2							
3							
4							
5							
6							
7							
8							
9							
10							
11							
Midnight							
1 a.m.							
2							
3							
4							
5							
6							
7							

Mention should be made of local diseases in and near the bladder
which affect control. Inflammation of the bladder, enlargement of the
prostate gland in men and prolapse of the uterus in women are among
disorders which cause bladder disturbances, and which can be improved
with treatment. Another type of bladder disturbance is that in which the
bladder seems to become paralysed and fills up with a very large amount
of urine. The patient may be dry for many hours then suddenly pass a
very large amount of urine without being aware of doing so.

Sometimes these patients develop *retention with overflow*. The bladder fills to a very large volume of urine and cannot be emptied, but small amounts of urine 'spill over' frequently although the bladder remains full. Patients with this trouble have 'dribbling incontinence'; they often cannot use a bedpan but may wet the bed when the pan is taken away. Although this conduct is very irritating to the nurse it is quite unintentional and it is due to disease not to mischievousness. It cannot be controlled by nursing measures, and often not even by medical treatment.

This brings us to the realization that while a very great deal can be done by good nursing to reduce the burden of incontinence, there are nearly always in a geriatric ward patients who are persistently incontinent. The majority of these have very extensive brain damage, and the mechanism responsible for controlling the bladder is injured beyond repair.

We turn therefore to considering what to do about established irreversible incontinence.

First the nurse must protect the patient's skin by not allowing it to remain in contact with urine. Once urine has left the body, one of its constituents is quickly decomposed by the action of bacteria into ammonia. This is a strong alkali which burns the skin and which has a powerful odour. So incontinent patients must be washed and changed immediately. Ordinary soap and water applied with a soft disposable cloth or tissue are adequate in most cases but sensitive skins should be cleansed with a cream, preferably one containing a small amount of acid.

Various types of incontinence pad may be used. The pads must be placed properly and they must be changed as soon as they are wet and before they begin to adhere to the patient's skin. At their best pads protect the bed rather than the patient. Some hospitals do not use them at all.

Incontinence Pants

Incontinence pants are of various designs but most of them consist of polythene pants secured by press-studs or ties with a pocket inside for insertion of an absorbent pad. They can be worn in conjunction with special underpants made of a 'one-way' fabric. These pants are of great value in protecting the patient's clothing, but the absorbent pads must be changed as soon as they are wet to protect the skin and to prevent odour.

Kanga Pants

A more recent development is pants made of a one way fabric with a waterproof pocket outside to hold an absorbent pad.

Incontinence appliances have been devised for use by male patients and are successful with some mentally alert men. They can so transform the life of such a person that they should always be tried. They work by collecting urine into a small bag worn around the genitals, from which the urine passes through a one-way valve and a tube to a larger storage bag. This can be worn inconspicuously beneath the trousers strapped on to the leg and can be emptied by releasing a tap at its lower end. (See page 72) The difficulty lies in ensuring a snug fit of the appliance around the genitals and preventing leakage of urine. This is particularly troublesome when the patient lies down. With careful attention to the selection of a suitable appliance and the method of wearing it these bags can be very helpful.

Catheterization

Catheterization is a last resort in the treatment of incontinence, except in the unconscious patient; the patient who has retention of urine with overflow, which cannot be dealt with in any other way; and the incontinent patient whose skin must be protected because of a burn, a pressure sore or a plaster close to the urethral orifice. Some geriatric units find that the easiest way to manage persistently incontinent patients is with a catheter and drainage bag; and if relatives learn to cope with this the patient can be sent home and looked after with the help of the District Nurse. This method is used only when other methods have failed and in the knowledge of the risks of urinary infection.

It must be avoided in those patients who cannot tolerate a catheter and who are likely to pull one out — even a balloon type catheter. Also many permanently catheterized patients eventually 'by-pass' the catheter, i.e. urine escapes along the side of it, in which situation he has the worst of both worlds.

11
The Bowels

Faulty action of the bowels is complained of by many old people. Some are pre-occupied with the subject and talk of little else. This concern with the bowels may have its origin in the patient's childhood, when a belief in the harmful effects of constipation was held much more strongly that it is today. The modern doctor or nurse may have a tendency to pooh-pooh a patient's reiterated complaint, but patients sometimes prove to be right in the end. Constipation and other bowel troubles cause considerable physical and mental distress and may lead to faecal incontinence or impacted faeces. So it is important to understand and attend to a patient's complaint of his bowels.

Pathological Physiology

In the normal young subject liquid faeces enters the colon at the ileo-caecal valve and progresses along the colon, becoming dried and bulky as it goes, until it reaches the rectum. When the faecal mass arrives at the rectum a signal is conveyed to the brain which registers a conscious sensation of fullness. This signal is sent on only one or two occasions each day, depending on the patient's habit; usually this is after meals, particularly after breakfast. This sensation is sometimes termed a 'call to stool'. The subject may answer the call by going to the toilet and defaecating; or he may suppress the call, in which case the sense of fullness disappears. It may not re-appear until many hours later and may then be stronger, but not necessarily so. In some cases the more often a call to stool is suppressed, the less obvious it is when it re-appears. The capacity of the brain of elderly people to be made aware of the presence of faeces in the rectum is much diminished. As a result they suffer from constipation: that is, the infrequent passage of firm faeces. Some geriatric patients accumulate large amounts of faeces, first in the rectum, then in the sigmoid colon or even higher up the bowel in the descending or transverse colon. Many of these patients usually complain bitterly of constipation although some are unaware of their trouble. The faeces can be felt in the left iliac fossa through the abdominal wall, and rectal examination reveals masses of rock-like faecal material distending the rectum. This condition is known as *faecal impaction.* It can reach such a severe degree that the lower bowel is obstructed. The patient suffers bouts of colicky abdominal pain as the colon attempts to drive faeces past the impaction, and he may even vomit and be admitted to a surgical ward as an acute abdominal emergency. For this reason doctors are taught the importance of never omitting a rectal examination in cases of suspected bowel obstruction, and indeed rectal examination should be performed routinely on admission in all geriatric patients. Another complication of faecal impaction is, paradoxically, diarrhoea. This may occur when liquid faeces from further up the bowel finds it way past the impacted mass of hard faeces in the lower bowel and trickles out. Faecal impaction may also be accompanied by faecal incontinence.

Lesser degrees of constipation may cause discomfort and anxiety but are not usually associated with diarrhoea or incontinence. Constipation may also lead to piles and fissures. In some cases the presence of a mass of faeces in the rectum interferes with the passage of urine and may contribute to the development of urinary retention. In some very ill bed patients a strange form of constipation occurs in which the rectum retains large quantities of soft almost liquid faeces which fail to dry in the usual way. The rectum cannot easily hold faeces in this moist condition and such patients are often incontinent of faeces.

Diarrhoea

This is a common disorder of old people. It may be caused by unsuitable diet, by bacteria, viruses and food poisoning and by many bowel diseases. The exact appearance of the faeces should be observed and reported. This information will assist the doctor to arrive at his diagnosis. The information required is:— the size, colour, odour, and consistency of the stool and the presence of blood, mucus and any unusual material. In the investigation of diarrhoea a specimen of the stool is sent to the laboratory or a swab is taken from high inside the rectum.

When more than one patient in the ward has diarrhoea at one time there is a suspicion of infectious disease or food poisoning and then collecting and culturing of all the bowel movements in the ward becomes necessary, while strict antiseptic precautions must be taken against the possible spread of the condition to other patients and staff.

Incontinence of faeces

One cause of incontinence of faeces associated with faecal impaction has already been described. Acute diarrhoea in a frail old person is another cause of incontinence. This is sometimes caused by injudicious purgation. The patient is incontinent simply because he cannot reach the toilet in time.

Incontinence of faeces associated with complete loss of control of the bowels is found mainly in very deteriorated long-term patients and most of them have severe brain damage involving among other parts, the area of the brain which controls the orderly evacuation of faeces.

Management

Before management of bowel disorders can be attempted it is important that accurate records of bowel function are made. It is not enough to ask the patient 'have your bowels moved today'? Even if he could tell you 'yes' or 'no' this information would be insufficient and many geriatric patients just wouldn't know.

Nursing staff must be trained to record and report on not just the number of bowel movements each patient has, but also the size, colour and consistency of the stool. This information should be recorded at some convenient place in the ward eg a blackboard on the sluice room wall.

The first step in the management of bowel disorders is the avoidance of constipation. Many patients believe that they become constipated because certain foods to which they are accustomed have been omitted from their diet. The hospital diet should provide plenty of fresh fruit and vegetables which provide 'bulk' and 'roughage', and when the patient expresses a preference for such presumed laxative foods as brown bread, porridge or 'all bran' he should be allowed these. Many patients put their faith in a glass of warm water first thing in the morning and this too should be allowed.

The details of toiletting should be carefully attended to. The patient should have an opportunity of defaecating at his regular time, which is usually before or after breakfast. He should rarely if ever be expected to defaecate into a bedpan as the acrobatic act required to maintain a precarious perch will leave no surplus energy for the act of evacuation. He must have warmth, comfort and *privacy* — the lack of these last inhibits the bowel of many a modest patient. He should not be left too long.

Physical and mental activity have beneficial effects on bowel regularity and the want of them promotes constipation. Once the patient is well and ambulant he is on the way to solving his bowel problem.

For those who cannot achieve regular evacuation of the bowel by their own unaided efforts some help is required.

Aperients

Many excellent preparations are on the market, and a little trial and error will determine the preparation and dose suitable for a given patient. It is best to use only two or three different preparations and these will be found to meet most needs. Liquid medicines are more acceptable than tablets and the dose can be more easily adjusted.

Suppositories

These are bullet-shaped pellets which are inserted deeply into the rectum as the patient lies on his left side with knees drawn up. They melt and release an active ingredient which stimulates the bowel directly and within fifteen to thirty minutes of insertion the patient experiences a powerful desire to defaecate. This method is quick and effective and for these reasons popular with patients and nurses. But some patients fail to retain the suppositories and others find their action too drastic.

Enemas

These act by distending the bowel with liquid and thus stimulating it to contract and to expel both the liquid and the retained faeces. It is not just a matter of flushing out the contents of the bowel. In the past it was usual for an enema to consist of a pint or more of soapy water inserted high up the bowel by a long nozzle and forced in by the effects of gravity.

This caused some old people to collapse and the method has been almost universally abandoned in favour of the modern small disposable enema. This contains 120ml of fluid in a plastic bag with nozzle attached which is merely squeezed into the rectum. The method is usually effective and rarely causes collapse. In more difficult cases a soap and water enema can be given. For patients with very hard faeces an enema of olive oil is instilled and the patient is asked to retain this for up to three hours if possible.

When other methods fail the nurse has to resort to *manual evacuation.* Unpleasant as this procedure is for nurse and patient alike it is very effective. In extreme cases of bowel obstruction due to massive faecal impaction it has been necessary to evacuate the bowel manually under general anaesthesia.

Diarrhoea

When associated with faecal impaction diarrhoea is cured by removal of the impacted faeces. Other forms of diarrhoea require *specific* treatment, ie removal of the cause and *symptomatic* treatment. Many drugs are used in an attempt to relieve the symptom of diarrhoea, of which the most effective are those which contain morphine in small quantity. For some of these morphine-containing preparations a Dangerous Drug prescription is not required, since the quantity of morphine is small, but nurses should none the less exercise great caution in their use.

Faecal Incontinence

The primary points in treatment are to ensure the patient's physical and mental health, to control the diet, to provide adequate opportunities for defaecation in privacy and comfort, to relieve faecal impaction and to control diarrhoea.

The most intractable problem is provided by the occasional very severely degenerated patient who smears faeces over his body and over the adjacent furniture. It is impossible to avoid the feeling of revulsion at this habit. It is due to extreme regression — ie the return to a primitive pattern of behaviour — and is not an indication of moral turpitude. This type of behaviour is found only in patients with very gross brain damage and often in the presence of faecal impaction, so at least that can be removed.

Faecal impaction is an ever present threat in geriatric patients. Even those who claim to be having regular bowel movements may be only half-emptying their rectum and retaining residual faeces. Accurate charting of bowel movements is necessary, so is constant vigilance and periodical rectal examination will reveal many surprises.

12
Care of the Patient in Bed

Only a small proportion of the patients in a geriatric ward require nursing in bed, but the needs of this group are heavy and they absorb much nursing time and effort. Some are being nursed through acute illness from which they can be expected to recover. Others are approaching the final stage of life. Some are sensible and continent, others are confused and incontinent.

The nurse's task is :

1   To nurse the patient in a comfortable position which must be changed regularly to prevent the breakdown of skin at pressure areas
2   To keep him fresh and clean by regular attention to face, hands, skin, oral hygiene and toilet needs
3   To ensure an adequate intake of nourishing food and fluid
4   To give all other necessary care and treatment

Positioning the Patient

The ill immobile patient requires frequent changes of position for his own comfort and to prevent pressure being exerted on the same parts of the body for long periods.

Many old people are more comfortable propped up — especially if they are suffering from heart or respiratory disease.

The position of an ill patient must be changed every two hours.

Lifting the Patient

All but the most ill patients should be lifted out of bed into a chair for bed making and on to a bedside commode for toilet purposes. For this, the nurse should use a patient-lifting device. When one is not available the following method of lifting is recommended:

Methods of Lifting a Patient in Bed

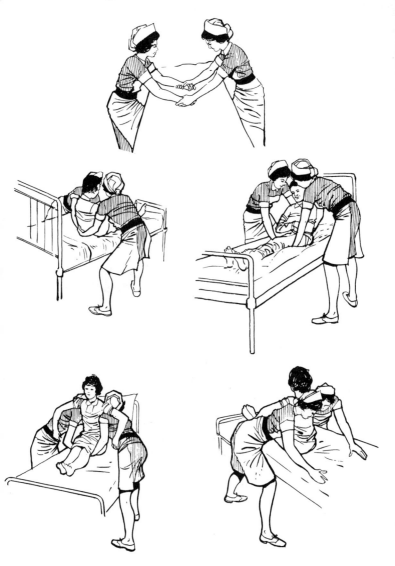

Prevention of Contracture

A contracture occurs when part of a limb is held in a faulty flexed position for a lengthy period. Eventually the muscles, ligaments, tendons and joint capsules become shortened and fibrosed and it is impossible to straighten them. This leads to severe disability. The following are some of the common forms of contracture together with the means of prevention.

Drop Foot

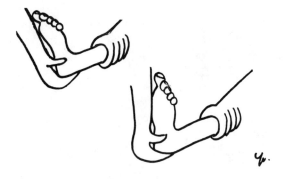

This occurs most readily when the foot is paralysed as in hemiplegia. Th may be aggravated by the weight of bed clothes, especially in a neatly made bed, pressing down on the foot. Drop foot can be prevented by the use of a foot cage, and by active dorsiflexion of the foot.
(See also foot cage on page 21)

Contracture of the Hip and Knee

This may occur in a spastic limb, as in hemiplegia, multiple sclerosis, or arthritis of the knee or hip and after fractures, eg of the neck of the femur, in the presence of pain. One still occasionally sees a condition which used to occur in the old workhouse days in which patients lie in the foetal position so bent that the knees touch their chins and the heels dig into the buttocks.

Contractures can be prevented by the relief of pain, the frequent correction of abnormal positions and the use of passive movement of the joint. The doctor may prescribe prone lying, sling suspension, or splintage of the affected limb, but the kind of patient who is liable to develop contractures is usually unable to tolerate these methods of treatment. Quadriceps exercises are given to maintain the tone and strength of the leg muscles.

Contracture of the Hand and Fingers

These occur in cases of hemiplegia and rheumatoid arthritis. In the latter condition, splints are required, and some cases need surgical correction. In hemiplegia the patient can be taught to do his own treat-

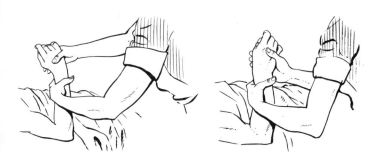

ment by extending the fingers of the paralysed hand using the good hand in abduction exercises of the thumb. Adduction deformity of the thumb makes it impossible for the patient to use the 'pinch-grip' function of the hand.

Contracture of Wrist, Elbow and Shoulders

The elbow and wrist are easily dealt with by putting them through their full range of movements at every opportunity. The shoulder is particularly liable to become contracted with loss of the abduction and extension movements necessary for dressing and this is partly because the weight of the unsupported arm drags on the joint capsule. The arm should therefore be supported on pillows and fully exercised whenever possible. The patient should be instructed to put the arm through its *full* range of movements for five minutes in every hour. Most patients are content to waggle the limb through the middle of the range only and this must be corrected.

Diet

The ill patient requires a nourishing diet to promote recovery and to prevent break down of body tissues. Many patients are unable to feed themselves; many have difficulty in swallowing. For some patients a semi-solid diet is the easiest one to take and this could consist of highly nutritious food reduced to a semi-solid state in a liquidizer, or alternatively tinned baby foods. A liquid diet is less easily taken and less tasty but is required for patients who have to be fed by tube. This should provide at least 1000 calories per day with up to 50G of protein, and is best given in the form of 'Complan'.

Fluid Intake
Ill old people often complain of thirst. Others become dehydrated without experiencing thirst. A daily fluid intake of 1500ml or more is usually required. The fluid intake and output should be charted. Fluids should be available at the bedside and staff and relatives should frequently offer fluids to the patient. An exception should be made of feeble patients with swallowing difficulties in whom inexpertly administered drinks may go down the wrong way into the trachea and be aspirated into the lungs. Only experienced staff should give drinks to these patients.

Oral Hygiene
Complaints of a dry tongue and a nasty taste in the mouth are common in most ill patients. A mouth-wash which is refreshing for a younger patient who can cope is not always advisable for an elderly person —

and never if the patient is mentally confused. Oral hygiene is best done with a moistened swab held by pressure forceps or wrapped round the index finger. Each swab is used once only. This mouth care should be done at 2–4 hourly intervals.

Oral Hygiene Tray

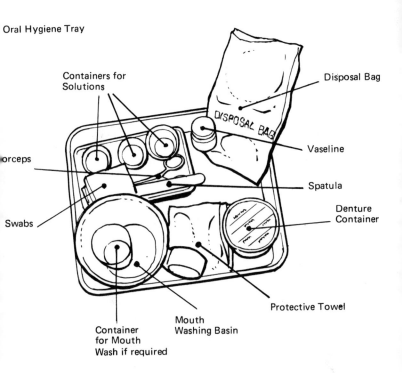

The patient is placed in a comfortable position. His upper garments are protected and when possible his co-operation gained. Remove dentures and inspect the mouth.

If the patient has his own teeth clean them regularly with his own toothbrush, in an up and down movement. Wrap a gauze swab round the blades of pressure forceps, fix securely and soak in cleansing lotion Sodium Bicarbonate 1 in 160 and clean the whole mouth in the followi manner changing the swab as often as necessary. A tongue depressor is often useful to control the movement of the tongue.

1. The tongue is cleaned first, with gentle strokes from side to side making sure the back of the tongue is clean. (Swabbing from back to front may cause the patient to retch).
2. Then the roof of the mouth and the floor if necessary.
3. Finally inside the cheeks and gums (food particles lodge here).

The swabbing of each part is repeated until the whole mouth is clean. If coating on the tongue is very adherent no attempt is made to peel it off as this might injure the surface of the tongue.

Care of the Skin

The principles of good skin care are cleanliness and avoidance of pressure and trauma.

Cleanliness

The ill patient requires to be bathed at least once a day.

In most cases he is too weak to be bathed in the bath and therefore must be bed-bathed.

Trolley with requirements for bathing in bed.

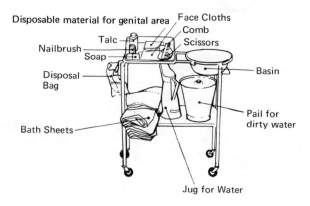

Disposable material for genital area — Face Cloths — Comb — Talc — Scissors — Nailbrush — Soap — Disposal Bag — Basin — Bath Sheets — Pail for dirty water — Jug for Water

Method of Bed-Bathing

A plentiful supply of hot water is brought to the bedside. The top bedclothes are removed and the top sheet replaced by a bath sheet. A bath sheet may also be placed under the patient to protect the bottom sheet from minor splashes. If a plastic mattress cover is in use then no other protection is necessary. Where special bathing sheets are not available then the patient must be given clean bed linen after bathing.

Heat of the Water

Body temperature is desirable but it can be made cooler if the patient wishes. Since nurse has to put her hands in the water there is little danger of it being too warm.

Washing Plan

The plan will depend very much on the degree of incapacity from which the patient is suffering. As little effort as possible should be expended by the patient. The face, neck, and ears are washed using a face cloth – with or without soap – as the patient wishes. If soap is used it should be thoroughly rinsed off. Since the face never feels dry unless when dried personally, the patient – if he is fit enough – should be allowed to do this.

Each arm in turn and the upper part of the body is now washed thoroughly, rinsed and dried taking great care to expose only the parts of the body being washed. Care must be taken to dry thoroughly under the arms and under the breasts in women. Moisture left here may causes sores to develop. If talcum powder is used it must be used sparingly – talcum mixed with sweat becomes gritty and is most uncomfortable.

If nurse has an assistant then she should help where necessary with washing and drying the patient in supporting the head or positioning the patient.

Using a different cloth or disposable material the genital area is then washed and dried.

To overcome the embarrassment this causes the patient he may be allowed to do this for himself.

Nurse must however ensure that the genital area is thoroughly dried.

Bed garments can now be replaced — fresh ones if necessary — and may be tucked up under the buttocks until the rest of the body is washed. To complete the bath fresh hot water is now used. Both limbs and feet are washed and dried thoroughly — especially between the toes. It is very refreshing and cooling for the patient confined to bed to have his feet washed by immersing them in a basin of warm water. Apply lanolin to any hard skin on feet or heels.

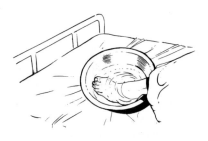

Provided that the patient is able to respond the safest way of ensuring that he is thoroughly dry is to ask him.

Nails should be cut after soaking when they are softer. Remember to cut nails straight across the tops of the toes. If the nails are too hard, or if the patient has poor blood circulation, no attempt should be made to cut them. The chiropodist will attend to this. Many women manicure their own finger nails — this they should be allowed to do — it often provides a morale booster.

After the Bath

After the patient has been bathed the bed is made with fresh linen if need be, and he is settled comfortably. Arrange his hair neatly and return toilet requisites to the locker. The screens can now be removed and windows re-opened. Soiled linen and water are now disposed of while the patient, now feeling refreshed, may want to sleep.

The trolley is cleaned and left ready for future use. While bathing the patient, the nurse should remember to observe the patient for any change in his physical and mental condition. Report these changes at once to sister.

Shaving Very Ill Patients

Nurse may have to shave a male patient who is too ill or weak to do this for himself and is distressed by the growth on his face. Most wards have an electric razor. In some hospitals there is a hospital barber who will shave the men regularly making the 'maintenance' shave easier for the nurse to manage.

Incontinent Patients

If incontinence of urine or faeces occurs the soiled areas should be washed as soon as possible with soap and warm water and dried thoroughly using disposable cloths or towels.

All wet or soiled linen should be removed.

The parts of the body on which pressure sores are likely to occur are shown below.

Prevention of Pressure and Trauma.

Position	DANGER AREAS						
1 Prone	Toes	Knees	Stomach	Elbows	Chin	Forehead	1
2 Recumbent	Heels	Buttocks	Small of back	Shoulders	—	—	2
3 Lateral	Heels	Inside knees	Hip	Shoulder	Ear Area	—	3

These are all points where the tissues are in danger of being compressed between the bed and the underlying bone. This pressure occludes the blood vessels of the area and interferes with its nutrition to such an extent that tissue death occurs. In the early stages of the pressure sore a red area is seen which remains red when the pressure is removed. This is a sign of great danger and intensive efforts must be made to prevent the advance of the condition. If this is not done, a blister may form, then th red area may turn black, the underlying tissue feels soft and boggy, and eventually the whole area breaks down, a slough is formed, pus and debris pour from it and the patient has a large and deep pressure sore. In other cases the damage is confined to the surface layer. The red area breaks, and a shallow circular saucer-shaped ulcer is left. This, unlike the large area of tissue necrosis, is often very painful, but it is far easier to heal. In addition it is possible for a small superficial but painful sore to be caused by tearing the skin. This may happen if a patient is dragged up the bed rather than lifted up — the friction between the sheet and the skin creates a shearing strain and tears off a small circle of skin from the underlying tissues.

Prevention of Pressure Sores

The basis of prevention of pressure sores is cleanliness, frequent turning and correct positioning. Equipment is a supplement to and not a substitute for a sound basic technique. Here are some points about vulnerable body parts:

Heels

Heel sores are easy to acquire, easy to avoid, difficult to cure and often very painful. Frequent change of position from back to side reduces the danger. So does prevention and treatment of oedema. Several types of heel pad are available to spread the load more widely. They are good provided the heel stays in them and provided the skin does not become excoriated by the sweat which these devices often generate.

A better method is to elevate the leg on a wedge pillow thus keeping the heel off the bed entirely.

124

Shoulder, Scapula, Ears

These and other parts of the body occasionally develop pressure necrosis but usually only in those patients who are extremely ill.

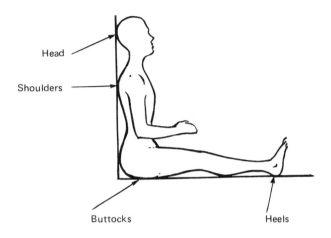

Head

Shoulders

Buttocks

Heels

Sacrum, Buttocks, Hips

These areas take the brunt of the body's weight and this is especially the case when the patient sits up. The best distribution of body weight is achieved when the patient lies flat with one pillow — but many patients have difficulty in tolerating this position.)

Patients 'at Risk'

Certain patients are more likely to develop pressure sores and these patients are termed to be 'at risk'. These are ill, immobile patients, poorly nourished or unable to take nourishment, incontinent, and often confused or demented patients.

These patients should be placed on a regular turning (see page 49). Each time the patient is turned the skin should be cleaned and dried. Reddened areas should be massaged (eg. with olive oil). The patient should be placed in the correct position on a clean sheet or drawsheet (without wrinkles or crumbs!!)

Items of Equipment

There are many items of equipment which will also help to relieve pressure.

Bed cages prevent the weight of bed-clothes on feet and ribs (pages 21, 116).

Different types of alternating pressure mattresses are designed to distribute the weight load in such a way that part of the body is relieved of pressure for frequent short intervals.

Pneumatress

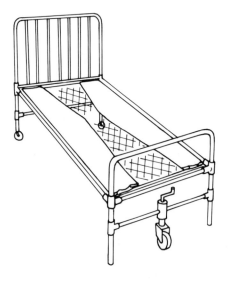

This consists of two durable inflatable air cells approximately six feet long and shaped to operate with maximum effectiveness at the three major pressure areas liable to bedsores. The air cells are positioned side

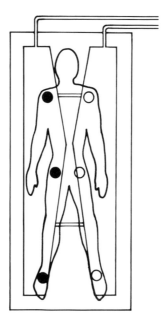

by side *beneath* the conventional mattress so that the patient's normal comfort is in no way impaired. Each cell is inflated independently by a compact silently operating pump which can be concealed beneath the bed or attached to the bed frame.

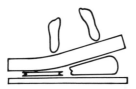

The effect is to raise gently first one side of the mattress to a maximum of six inches, over a 15 minute period, deflate and repeat the procedure on the other .

Ripple-Bed

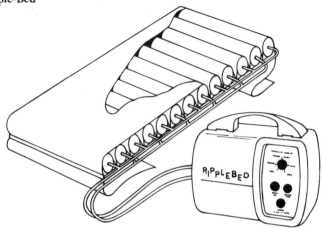

In a ripple bed — the large cell type being best — alternate cells are inflated and deflated at frequent intervals.

Sheepskins

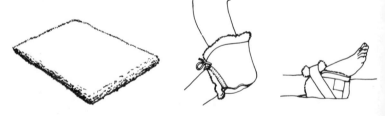

Sheepskin can be used for protective mats and for protecting specific joints and areas.

Cubex Pads
Available in various sizes, the pads are filled with shifting polystyrene beads so that they will easily mould to the patient's body. Thus pressure will be distributed over the largest possible surface. Even slight moveme

on the part of the patient will stimulate the blood circulation of the skin through a slight massaging action.

Treatment of Pressure Sores

The principles of treatment of an established sore are:

1 Prevention of further local pressure
2 Prevention of contamination by urine, faeces, sweat
3 Elimination of dead tissue
4 Control of infection
5 Treatment and mobilization of the patient

Removal of dead tissue is essential to allow exposure of the healing surfaces. Dead tissue is called *slough*. It may be adherent or fairly loose. It may be soft and yellow or hard and black. Sometimes it forms a dense black crust over the whole area of the sore; sometimes it is present only at the edge of an otherwise healing ulcer.

Adherent slough needs to be cut away by the doctor using a scalpel and forceps. This is painless, as the knife cuts through tissues which have no nerve endings, so no local anaesthetic is required. Looser dead tissue can often be pulled away with forceps while the ulcer is being dressed. Dead tissue which is not suitable for removal in either of these ways can be eased off gradually by the use of certain ointments, creams or sprays, of which the best known are 'Aserbine' and 'Elase'. These act slowly over a period of days by dissolving the dense fibres by which the dead tissue is attached.

Sometimes dead tissue comes away more readily in the bath. The presence of bedsores is no contra-indication to the patient having a bath; indeed a bath is very beneficial and comforting, since it removes pressure and promotes circulation, as well as rinsing the ulcer. A mild antiseptic such as Savlon should be added to the bath water, and the bath should be washed down with antiseptic solution after use. Patients with pressure sores can be bathed twice daily if possible.

Control of infection is required before a sore can heal, otherwise tissue destruction proceeds, with great pain. Infection is recognised by suppuration in the sore and redness and swelling of the surrounding skin. This should be reported to the doctor, who may prescribe an antibiotic to be given by mouth or injection. Local treatment consists of removing pus by frequent changes of dressings, and by the use of antiseptics and antibiotics in the form of a liquid solution or spray preferably, although if suppuration is not excessive a cream or ointment may be preferred. Useful preparations include:

Hibitane solution or cream.
Anaflex paste
Terra-cortril ointment.

There are very many others. Each nurse has her own favourite, and it is preferable to use only a small range of preparations and to become familiar, through experience, with the best way to use them. But we should remember that the only purpose of local treatment is to eliminate infection with the minimum disturbance to the natural process of healing. There appears to be no justification for applying to an ulcer such substances as dried milk powder, cod liver oil, dried plasma, honey and oxygen, all of which seem to be used quite widely.

If a large sore is healing very slowly despite the elimination of infection it may be possible to achieve healing more rapidly by the use of skin grafting.

Treatment and mobilisation of the patient promotes healing of sores. Patients with pressure sores need a high protein diet. If they are reluctant to eat they should receive extra milk drinks fortified with 'Complan' or 'Carnation Instant Breakfast Food' or similar powdered high protein preparations. Anaemia is treated by an iron preparation if appropriate, and sometimes by blood transfusion. Once the patient can get up and move about, thereby removing pressure and promoting circulation, sores heal rapidly.

The prevention and treatment of pressure sores requires regular and persistent care by the nurse using the most skilful and meticulous nursing techniques. With geriatric patients the prevention and treatment of pressure sores is not solely the responsibility of the nurse. The knowledge and experience of the doctor is also required.

13

Confusion and Behavioural Disturbances

One of the more worrying, perplexing, and perhaps frightening aspects of geriatric nursing is dealing with patients who are mentally disturbed. Especially is this so for the inexperienced nurse on night duty.

Yet the nurse who has once learned how to handle such patients can find their management very gratifying.

But first an explanation is required of the reasons for old people's behaviour becoming disturbed.

Mental Confusion

The term 'mental confusion' is used to describe these conditions in which the patient's thinking power is disturbed. Confused patients are often described as disorientated for time, place, or persons; that is they do not know where they are, what time, day, month, or year it is; and who the people are around them. They may have no idea at all about these matters or, more commonly, they have incorrect ideas.

For example they may believe that they are at home or at work rather than in hospital; they may believe it is daytime in the middle of the night; they may be under the impression that the nurse is their daughter.

Characteristically this confusion is a fluctuating condition. At times the patient may be quite lucid, at other times severely disturbed. Their disorientation may affect their behaviour. For example they may insist on getting out of bed in the middle of the night to put their clothes on in the belief that it is time to get up and go out to work. Confused patients are often quite intelligent. Their speech and behaviour develops logically from their beliefs about where they are: it is only the beliefs themselves that are awry.

Confused patients can be perfectly quiet, or they can be extremely noisy. When this happens it may be because they are bewildered, frightened, and frustrated. For example a patient once struck another patient, and it was only later discovered that he had thought that the other patient was his father, and he became extremely angry when the latter failed to answer his questions and showed no signs of recognition.

Confusion has many causes and can occur at all ages. A confused state occurs in association with infectious diseases such as pneumonia or meningitis even in young patients when it is called delirium.

In elderly patients confusional states are particularly liable to complicate infectious diseases and anoxic states like asthma. They are also found in cases of congestive cardiac failure, myocardial infarction, renal failure, dehydration, thyroid disease, some forms of anaemia, liver disease, alcoholism and many other conditions.

Confusional states may be brought on by drugs- notably barbiturates, narcotics, hypnotics, tranquillizers, anti-Parkinsonism drugs, digoxin, and others.

Characteristically a confusional state clears up quickly when the cause has been removed, and the patient becomes mentally normal again. This usually takes only a few days. Trouble may occur if the patient is heavily sedated to prevent him being restless and noisy. The sedative drug itself may worsen the confusion or it may sedate the patient so much that his fluid intake is reduced which further aggravates the condition. The presence of pain, a full bladder, or a loaded rectum may also worsen the confusional state.

The prime point in the management of mental confusion in old people is to identify the cause and eliminate it by treating and curing infection; administering oxygen; clearing the bowel; etc.

The next essential is to avoid doing anything which might aggravate the situation and do try not to use powerful sedative drugs until you see whether the patient can be calmed by a cup of tea, a cigarette, or a small alcoholic drink.

It is also important not to argue with the patient, not to attempt to reason with him, because his befuddled brain cannot think reasonably.

Rather he should be humoured and calmed, and the whole object of the nurse's handling of the patient should be to keep the emotional temperature down. The restless patient should not be forced back to bed the frightened patient should not be further frightened by being told that he will fall.

This advice is easier to give than to act upon but it is the right advice. The test of a good nurse is the ability to calm, soothe, and relieve the frightened, noisy, confused old patient − but when the simpler measures which have been advocated do not work medical help is required.

The following simulated situation will demonstrate clearly how a good nurse might handle such a patient.

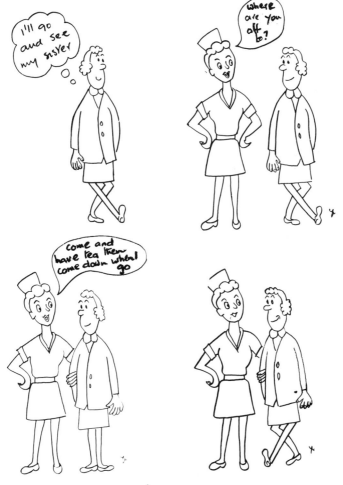

A calm end to a temporary upset.

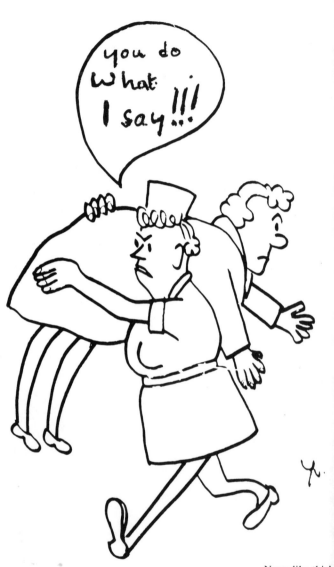

Never like this!

Dementia

The human brain is a remarkable organ capable of controlling the intricate movements of the acrobat, performing the abstruse calculations of the mathematician, creating the noble works of the artist.

It performs these and a million more humdrum functions by using an enormous bank of nerve cells (neurones) linked together by an intricate network of connections. Each of these nerve cells is unique and irreplaceable. From early middle age the cells begin to wear out and die. This is why many people long before they reach old age find their memory and concentration are not what they used to be.

Old people have many fewer brain cells than they had in their youth but are still capable of leading normal lives and even of taking active parts in politics or creative writing.

But in some unfortunate old people the loss of brain cells is much more rapid and they reach old age with insufficient cells remaining intact to enable them to cope with the demands made upon them. The brain is — as it were short-staffed.

We call this condition of excessive loss of brain cells dementia.

One type of dementia is due to disease in the arteries bringing blood to the brain. These have blocked and the cells which they supplied are starved to death. This is known as arteriosclerotic dementia.

There are however other types of dementia which are not due to arterial disease.

Dementia is a common disease. Perhaps about 5% of old people suffer from some degree of dementia.

The commonest age of onset is in the middle seventies but it may begin earlier or later. Females are more often affected than males.

The condition often manifests itself gradually. For a long time the relatives may notice nothing unusual at all or may merely comment that the patient is forgetful, but no more than they believe might be expected of that age. Then something happens which alarms them- the patient wanders out and gets lost, or burns out a kettle because she has forgotten to turn off the gas tap. When examined by a doctor the patient is found to have quite severe dementia.

The characteristic symptom is loss of memory for recent events. Patients do not seem to take in things that have just happened, or what they have just been told. The event or the statement fails to register on their memory and is instantly forgotten. Relatives find that they have to tell them the same thing over and over again. They lose things because they forget where they have put them. But although the patients are deprived of what we call short term memory they retain their memory for more distant events. They remember things that happened in their childhood but not what occurred five minutes ago. They also remember words, phrases and ideas which they have known for a long time and are able to carry on an intelligent conversation. They remember a familiar environment and regular patterns of behaviour. In favourable circumstances they may thus be able to function fairly normally. We can say that demented patients are not necessarily confused.

But if a demented patient takes ill – for example with heart failure – and he has to be admitted to hospital an entirely different situation results.

Because of his loss of short-term memory he quickly forgets the circumstances leading up to his admission to hospital. He cannot identify the people around him and cannot take in what they are telling him.

He thus very quickly becomes disoriented for time, place, and persons and so he becomes confused. And because underlying his confusional state he has a brain that is already abnormal it is much more difficult for him to regain normal orientation once the acute episode has settled down than it is for the undemented patient.

Because of their limited intellect demented patients in hospital are not too difficult to deal with. They do not in general become agitated or frightened. They forget their problems quickly, and accept their situation contentedly. Indeed they are often happy people.

The opposite is the patient who has a tendency to restless wandering in search of something which he cannot describe, who is continually being brought back to the ward and is continually off on the move again. Such patients require an enclosed area where they can walk without endangering themselves.

Some demented patients have accompanying disturbances of balance, of bladder and bowel function. Many do not, and can be among the 'healthiest' patients in a geriatric ward.

It should be apparent that drug treatment cannot influence dementia. Indeed drugs by interfering with the action of the remaining brain cells are positively harmful and are best avoided.

The following table summarises the differences between Confusion and Dementia.

Dementia	Confusion
A disease characterised by a loss of brain cells.	A symptom due to disturbed function of brain cells.
Commonest in old age	Can occur at any age but is common in old age.
Caused by brain disease	Brought on by disease outwith the brain.
Permanent and irreversible	Temporary and reversible.
Impaired short-term memory	Short-term memory may be impaired.
Few lucid periods	Lucid periods are common
Behaviour not necessarily disturbed	Behaviour often affected

Other Psychological Disturbances

These types of psychological disturbances are sometimes found in geriatric patients.

Depression

This is common and many old patients have a lot to be depressed about. When one considers the losses they have suffered — loss of health, loss of income, loss of a life partner, loss of children, loss of status and role in society — the wonder is that more of them are not depressed.

A goodly number of geriatric patients are perfectly ready to admit that they are ready to die and would be happy to do this, but the number who actually attempt suicide is small.

But it is unwise to be complacent and even the very old can and do make determined suicide attempts.

Depression is caused more by physical illness than by social and psychological factors mentioned above, and most old people would accept their lot contentedly if they had their health.

Loss of eyesight and hearing are particularly hard to bear and the sense of being a burden to others is a particularly potent cause of depression. Patients who live alone are probably less vulnerable in this respect.

Religious faith sustains many old people through great hardships.

Paranoid Illness

Mild degrees of paranoia are occasionally seen when old people complain that they have been poisoned, blame others irrationally, feel everything goes wrong, or make wild allegations about each other.

This can be hard to bear when nurses are accused of cruelty, theft, or promiscuity unless the patient's mental state is appreciated.

Anxiety

Anxiety is a very common symptom in old age, and may be manifested by attention-seeking behaviour in which the patient demands special attention to himself at the expense of everyone else in the ward. Such patients can be hard to put up with but it is often possible to find out what is causing the anxiety — it may be fear of cancer, worry about wetting a bed, concern for a relative.

But such patients usually have a worrying nature, and allaying their anxiety on one score merely sets them off worrying about something else.

Old people are really just young people grown old. In their behaviour in a ward they display all the facets of human behaviour, and the good nurse will find endless fascination in observing them and much scope for exercising sympathy, kindness and insight.

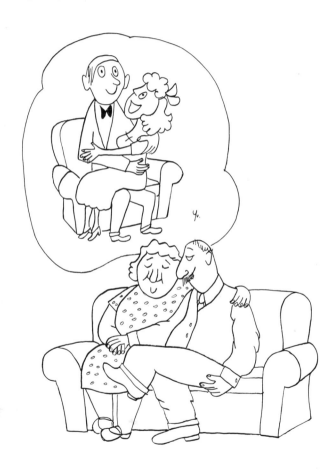

14
Drug Administration

Geriatric patients often have a number of different diseases at once so that doctors require to use a number of drugs to relieve them.

The pouring of many powerful chemical substances into an old person's body may be highly beneficial but sometimes things go wrong.

Drugs may have considerable side effects because elderly patients may be unduly sensitive to them.

Routes of Administration

S.C.	Subcutaneous
I.M.	Intramuscular
I.V.	Intravenous
S.L.	Sublingual

In the administration of drugs the nurse's aim should always be that the correct patient

receives the correct dose

of the correct drug

at the correct time

The drug, dose, and time of administration should be clearly written up by the doctor and signed by him.

The nurse should ascertain the drugs each patient should receive, their dosages, and times of administration from an order previously printed out and signed by a doctor.

The individual patient's prescription sheet is commonly used and meets this need.

There is also a space to record the date each drug is commenced, the date of discontinuation and the initials of the doctor discontinuing it.

Drugs should always be given from a written instruction signed by a doctor and not from a verbal order.

Drug Prescription Sheet

Sheet No.			PRESCRIPTION SHEET														

DRUGS BY INJECTION – REGULAR PRESCRIPTIONS.

Date Comm.	DRUG (Block Letters)	DOSE	TIMES OF ADMINISTRATION								METHOD OF ADMIN.	SIGNATURE	DISCONTINUED	
			AM 8	AM 10	MD 12	PM 2	PM 6	PM 10	MN 12	Other Times			DATE	INITIALS
A														
B														
C														
D														
E														

OTHER DRUGS – REGULAR PRESCRIPTIONS

F														
G														
H														
I														
J														
K														
L														
M														

DRUGS BY INJECTION – ONCE ONLY PRESCRIPTION.   **DIET**

DATE GIVEN	DRUG (Block Letters)	DOSE	TIME OF ADMIN.	METHOD OF ADMIN.	SIGNATURE	GIVEN BY INITIALS	DATE	DETAILS	INITIALS

OTHER DRUGS – ONCE ONLY PRESCRIPTIONS

WARD	NAME OF PATIENT	AGE	UNIT NUMBER	CONSULTANT

The nurse in a geriatric ward should administer the medicines in the usual way taking the necessary care and precautions. With old people however, she may meet the following difficulties:

1   The patient may have difficulty in swallowing tablets or capsules.

The drug can then be given in alternative liquid form or the tablet can be crushed inside a piece of tinfoil (so that no part of the dosage is lost) and then mixed with something palatable—eg honey or jam.

2   The patient pretends to swallow the tablet but doesn't!

The nurse must stay with the patient until she is definitely certain the tablet has been swallowed.

3 The patient refuses to take the medicine

It may again be possible to mix the drug with food, or in a drink — but remember the whole of the food or the drink has to go over!! Nurse will require all her powers of persuasion.

If the patient cannot or will not take the medicine ordered this should be reported to the sister or doctor.

The drug may then need to be given by another route, either intramuscularly or intravenously — particularly if the patient is very ill.

No. 1031

DATE	6 a.m.	10 a.m.	12 md.	2 p.m.	6 p.m.	10 p.m.	12 mn.	OTHER TIMES			COMMENTS ON DISCREPANCIES

WARD   NAME   UNIT   NUMBER   DRUG RECORDING SHEET

REGULAR PRESCRIPTIONS

PLEASE ENTER APPROPRIATE CODE FROM THE BURDEN SHEET

A drug record sheet on which nurse records when a drug has been given and initials each entry is a useful check that drugs have been administered correctly. This is particularly important in a geriatric ward where patients are up and about and so the medicine round is not really a simple tour of patients in bed without interruption.

15
Accidents and their Prevention

Accidents are a major cause of illness and death in the elderly and aged, because of their diminished perception of the environment and their delayed reactions to danger, combined with their social isolation and their need to live in a society geared to the needs of a younger more active population. For example the old person in the bus may be slow to realise that his stop has been reached; he is jostled as he attempts to reach the exit; he is afraid that the bus will drive away before he is able to leave it; he may fail to perceive the kerb — so he trips and falls. One of the reasons for admitting some old people to homes and hospitals is to protect them from the dangers to which they may be lead by their physical and mental frailty.

In hospital old people are never left alone, yet accidents still occur. Nurses must learn to think in terms of the possibility of accidents and be constantly vigilant to prevent them. Each time an accident occurs the exact circumstances should be studied, so that another accident will not occur from the same source.

The accidents to be discussed are:

1 *Falls*
    (a)   in and around the bed
    (b)   in the ward and day room area
    (c)   in the toilet
    (d)   in the bath
2 *Burns and Scalds*
3 *Swallowing and Choking*

A section on fits is included in this chapter.

Falls

After a fall it may be difficult to reconstruct the exact sequence of events since the patient may be confused and there may have been no witness.

Falls in and around the Bed

Restless patients may fall out of bed and require to have cot sides to prevent this accident. Most patients who need cot sides appreciate the security which these give, but some, particularly the confused, resent them and may attempt to climb over them and may fall in this way. Many patients found lying on the floor beside their bed have not actually fallen out of bed. They have tried to get out of bed by themselves when unfit to do so, and have fallen while attempting this feat, or at the stage of sitting up or trying to stand at the bedside. Patients often make these misguided attempts during the night when they need the toilet and are dulled by sleep or sedatives. While prevention by observation and exhortation is the best cure it is impossible in a busy ward to keep watch all the time. So two helpful rules are always to ensure that if the bed has wheels the brakes are on; (some patients fall because they lean against an unbraked bed which rolls away from them) and to place a stout chair at the bedside to give the patient support.

Falls in the Ward and Day Room Area

A weak patient may fall in the ward or day room when trying to rise from his chair or as a result of sitting down too heavily in the chair which topples beneath him. Another cause of falls is standing up from a sitting down position on a wheelchair, the brakes of which are not properly applied.

Unsteady patients should always be accompanied when walking. But even steady ones fall if they encounter a loose end of linoleum or carpet or a slippery floor. Badly dressed patients trip over slippers or dressing gowns. These external hazards must be avoided.

Falls in the Toilet

Falls in the toilet are particularly serious because the patient may strike his head against a hard surface. Unsteady patients should not be left alone in the toilet. Falls may be caused by dizziness brought on by sleepiness or sedatives, by straining to pass urine or faeces, or by the sudden change of posture or temperature. A wet and slippery floor is an added hazard.

Falls during Bathing

Falls during bathing should rarely occur since geriatric patients are not left to bathe alone. Non-slip bath mats and well-placed hand-grips reduce the chance of accidents.

Apart from falls due to *extrinsic* causes, such as tripping over a carpet, many falls have an *intrinsic* cause. These falls are often called 'drop attacks' and they characteristically come as a surprise to the patient. His usual account of the fall is 'I was just walking to the day room when my legs seemed to give way under me and down I went". These falls are not preceded by dizziness or loss of consciousness, but often the patient has difficulty in rising after the fall. The exact cause of drop attacks is not understood, but they are thought to have something to do with a temporary loss of balance function. Another common type of fall is brought on by a rapid rotating head movement, for example by a patient suddenly turning to look over his shoulder. The spinning movement is too much for the body's balance system and down he goes. Also many diseases in geriatric patients are associated with disturbance of balance, notably strokes, Parkinson's disease and any disease causing weakness of the legs. Finally some old people fall because of visual disturbances and one cause to be remembered is the use of bifocal lenses — many an old person misjudges distances, particularly when going downstairs, because he fails to allow for the distortion caused by these spectacles.

When a patient falls the nurse should immediately check that there is no bleeding and no obvious fracture. If she is in any doubt she should immediately summon the doctor. Otherwise the patient is put to bed and kept warm because a fall can cause a drop in body temperature. The doctor must in any case always be notified of the accident. Fracture of the neck of the femur can occur with great ease in an ill old person even after quite a trivial fall and often without very obvious clinical signs. Any injured part should be inspected daily for some time after the fall to see if delayed bruising occurs.

Burns and Scalds

Most burning accidents in the house are associated with cooking or the use of paraffin, gas, electric or open coal fires. The hospital patient is free of these hazards. Nor is he likely to be burned by an electric blanket or hot water bottle, because all nurses know that these can be very dangerous if left with an old person who may not perceive the degree of heat or may not be able to withdraw the threatened limb from the source of heat. Hospital patients are often burned by cigarettes which fall out of their hands into their clothing or bedclothes (old people pay scant regard to hospital regulations on this subject). They are sometimes scalded by hot tea or soup spilling on to their chest, when they feed themselves in bed.

In the event of a burning accident the nurse will take immediate action to prevent the spread of the fire in accordance with the instructions she has been given on fire prevention in her hospital. If garments are on fire the fire must be instantly extinguished by smothering with a blanket or rolling on to the ground. The burned parts of the body should be immediately immersed in cold water and kept there until help in dealing with the situation can be summoned.

Scalding accidents in the bath or shower should never occur, since careful testing of water temperature is an essential part of the procedure. A patient can burn himself by accidentally touching the tap, or in some types of shower the sudden drop in the cold water pressure with normal hot water pressure and the absence of mixing valve may cause a sudden rise in water temperature. The first aid treatment of scalds is also immediate and prolonged immersion of the scalded part in cold water.

Swallowing and Choking

A piece of bread or meat becomes stuck in a patient's throat. This is a real emergency and the patient is in immediate danger of death due to asphyxia. The nurse must act at once, there is no time to wait for a doctor to be summoned. She should remove the patient's dentures and put her hand right down the throat and pull the food out; then immediately turn the patient on his face, raise the foot of the bed and thump his back until he coughs up further food fragments and mucus. Then the doctor should be summoned to extract any remaining food, to aspirate secretions and to take any further necessary action.

All frail patients should have meat and similar food cut into small portions before it is served to them.

Most accidents are due to human failings in patients and mechanical failing in equipment.

Learn from experience. Find out what went wrong every time an accident occurs, and don't let the same thing happen a second time.

Fits and 'Turns'

The nurse may witness various kinds of fits in geriatric patients most of these of very short duration. She may be the only one to see what happened and she can be of great help to the doctor by describing exactly what she observed.

Here are some questions a nurse should ask herself:

1 What was the patient doing when the 'fit' or 'turn' commenced, eg lying in bed, sitting in a chair, getting up, standing or walking, eating, micturating, defaecating

2 Did he lose consciousness? If so for how long?

3 Was he rousable, eg by touching the eyelashes or by applying pressure on the orbit?

4 Were there abnormal movements? If so what parts of the body moved and for how long?

5 Did he have a warning; if so what exactly did he say and do?

6 Did he fall, if so which came first the fall or the 'turn'?

7 Did he become pale or flushed?

8 Did he vomit?

9 Did he complain of a visual disturbance?

10 Did he pass urine or faeces?

11 What happened to his pulse — was it rapid, slow or absent, regular or irregular, strong or weak?

12 What was his blood pressure?

Of the many different kinds of turn that can occur the commonest is *syncope* which is really just a simple faint. The patient's appearance may be deathly and he may remain unconscious for longer than usual in younger people, but he will recover completely. He should be immediately laid in bed with head down and his pulse and blood pressure should be charted initially every five minutes and then less often. Epileptic attacks are also quite common and the usual steps should be taken of removing the dentures or inserting a gag between the teeth. Patients with change of heart rate or rhythm may require immediate medical measures and a doctor should be informed forthwith.

6
Terminal Care

The material to be presented here is a discussion of the questions which face doctors and nurses who care for the dying. No one can lay down what is right and what is wrong. It can be helpful to discuss the subject between the medical and nursing staff, the chaplain and the social worker.

The following questions are discussed here:

1 Do patients know when they are going to die?
2 What should they be told?
3 What should their relatives be told?
4 What treatment should be given to the dying patient?
5 What is the role of the chaplain?

In the majority of deaths in geriatric units the patients do not know that they are going to die. Death is preceded by weeks or months of diminishing cerebral function and failing understanding of the environment. In these cases of progressive dementia the patient also loses his awareness of his own body and experiences little of the pain or discomfort which would be felt by a patient with intact mind and similar bodily disabilities. Dementia as it were, tempers the wind to the shorn lamb. In such cases telling the patient or the relatives presents no problems. The one does not grasp what is said, the other does not require to be told the obvious.

If such patients experience an acute illness like pneumonia or heart failure in a very late stage of their progressive dementia, what should be done for them? There are three views.

One is that they must be treated as thoroughly as would any other patient at any other age with the same disease.

A second view is that their life should not be needlessly prolonged and all treatment should be withheld.

A third opinion is that it is mandatory upon the doctor and nurses to take any steps which might increase the *comfort of the patient* and in some cases this may well include the use of antibiotics and other potentially life-saving measures, but that prolongation of life for its own sake is not required of the doctor.

Which of these views is held is a matter of individual conscience, but it is of value for this problem to be aired and for people who work together to reach a consensus in their actions or at least a respect for one another's sincerely held views.

A minority of geriatric patients experience great bodily and mental distress in the period preceding their death. Many are weary of this world, of the burden of their own suffering and of being, as they believe, a source of trouble to others. It matters little whether their forthcoming death is due to cancer or to any other condition (indeed many diseases from which the old suffer are more painful and more distressing than cancer). Many of these patients will confess, if directly questioned on the subject that they pray to God each day to take them away. But the patient's estimate of his state may be wrong. He is ill, depressed and pessimistic and in this state he sees death as the only escape from his torment. But he may never have been properly investigated or treated and it may well be that he can be relieved of much of his suffering by proper treatment. Will he then still want to die? The fact that a patient wants to die should lead to an intensification rather than to a cessation of medical endeavour.

What of the patient who is manifestly dying, who remains mentally alert and who does not seem to be aware of how ill he is? He may have cancer; perhaps he has undergone surgery and radiotherapy and has every reason to suspect his fate, yet he seems to remain unaware of the nature of his illness and does not even appear to be unduly concerned. A few of these patients ask what is wrong with them, most do not. Some doctors believe that patients should be told what is wrong with them and at the same time should be reassured that a great deal can be done for them. In this way, they feel, people will gradually get rid of their natural fears. Others believe that patients play a game with their doctors in which each pretends that the other does not know what the matter is, thus neatly avoiding discussion of a painful topic, and it would be breaking the rules of the game if one or other were to 'tell'. A third view is that the dying patient's greatest possession is hope. It does not matter how slender that hope is, he will clutch on to it and no one should deprive him of it. In this view the dying patient should be encouraged to believe that he is getting on well, despite all evidence to the contrary, and any little white lie which will strengthen his belief is to be accepted.

No one can tell a nurse how to behave in the presence of a dying patient and a good nurse does not need to be told, since she will treat him exactly as she treats all other patients. It would be unthinkable for her to speak heartlessly in his presence, but the adoption of a frivolous approach should be equally unacceptable. Humour is more appreciated than solemnity at the bedside of the dying provided the patient's reaction is assessed. Excessive attention may alarm the patient.

In speaking to relatives one never forgets that the loss of a spouse or parent in advanced old age is a grievous blow to the bereaved.

After the death they need no reminding that the patient lived a full span of life; but while he is still alive they have the same strong urge to cling to him as at any other age. After all they have never known what life is like without him. The majority of relatives of dying old people are very understanding, make few demands on the nurses and express grateful appreciation of what is being done. There are always some 'difficult' relatives, and the good nurse makes allowances for the emotional strains to which they are exposed. Dying old people to whom religion is a strong force will welcome a visit from a minister of religion or priest, and there is no need to worry about their being frightened by this. Even many of those with no formal religious affiliation derive benefit from a talk with the chaplain.

The enormous problems associated with the last period of life have been touched upon here only very briefly. We do not know whether our actions for dying patients have brought comfort or unhappiness. We must only remember that all that we say and do is observed and interpreted by our patients. The rest is for the individual conscience to decide.

17
Nursing in the Day Hospital

The Day Hospital is a part of the service which a geriatric unit gives to the community.

It is a separate part of the geriatric unit which is as a rule open from 9 am–5 pm from Monday till Friday.

It provides the following functions:

1 The investigation and treatment of elderly patients who are being well cared for at home but who might benefit from the treatment and social activities of the department

2 The maintenance treatment of patients recently discharged from the wards who have not yet completed the transition to full independence at home

3 The periodic care of dependent patients whose relatives require temporary relief — even for a few hours a week — from the constant strain of caring for them

4 The investigation and rehabilitation of special 'high risk' groups of old people

eg the very elderly

those who live alone

those recently bereaved etc

Organization of the Day Hospital

The day hospital may be a converted ward or unused building in the hospital or it may have been specially built for the purpose. Usually has from 15 to 40 patients a day. Most of them are brought to the day hospital by ambulance or mini bus. On their arrival the patients are settled in, taken to the toilet, given a cup of tea and started on their activities. New patients are seen by a doctor; so are others at regular intervals. They may be sent for X-ray, blood tests and other investigations. Some require nursing procedures such as dressings, injections, suppositories or enemas. The majority have individual or group physiotherapy, occupational therapy and speech therapy. After a busy morning's work, they go to the toilet again; have lunch and are allowed rest. In the afternoon they may have further treatment or else they may be given recreational activities which include playing games, crafts and hobbies, listening to music, singing or a percussion band. Then afternoon tea is served and transport comes to take them home.

In the course of the day patients are seen by the chiropodist, the medical social worker, perhaps the chaplain, staff from the ward where they were hospitalized and members of voluntary organizations. They can be put in touch with agencies and clubs outside the hospital. When they no longer need to attend the day hospital they are transferred to the community again.

An important part of the organization is to trace who has failed to attend and to find out why.

The staff of the day hospital usually comprises a Sister-in-charge, assisted by trained nurses, auxiliaries, domestic staff and a clerkess/transport officer. Usually the doctors, rehabilitation staff and social workers come from the geriatric unit, whose staff must be increased accordingly. Their work is enriched by the varied experience and the continuity of care. Voluntary workers are generous in coming forward to help in the day hospital, especially as aides to the physiotherapist and occupational therapist and in the games and crafts work. A special need is for someone to be available to check usually by a home visit on those who fail to attend.

Nursing in the Day Hospital

The regular hours of work are an attraction to married nurses. The work itself is of great interest but the nurse requires to adapt herself to the very special demands that will be made on her. Technical nursing is only a small part of her work. Much of what she has to do is administrative — seeing that the right patient is in the right place at the right time. Another part is 'mothering' — seeing that patients have their likes and dislikes attended to, that they are not overtired or in need of the toilet or sitting in a chair they dislike. Another part of their work is listening to what the patient has to say about his health, his home, his family, deciding whether he is well and happy or whether something more needs to be done.

A large part of the nurse's day is spent on 'jollying along' her patients, cheering them up, seeing that they have a good time, that they return home from the Day Hospital feeling the better for it.

More than half of the geriatric units in the United Kingdom now have Day Hospitals. Some pupil nurses may have had experience of working in these units. All should have the opportunity of visting one. They will be impressed by the atmosphere of hope and vitality which pervades them. Day Hospitals for geriatric patients are a new feature of the British hospital scene. Their success ensures them a permanent place.

18
Nursing the Old Person at Home

In the course of her training the pupil nurse may have the opportunity of accompanying a District Nurse on her visits. She will find this very different from the conditions and situations with which she has become accustomed in hospital.

The most obvious difference is the lack of the familiar essential equipment — the hospital bed, the bed-side locker, the overbed table and so on. Together with this is the encumbrance of domestic furniture and floor coverings, leaving little room for manoeuvre. The situation calls for ingenuity and improvisation. A cage to protect the feet against the pressure of bedclothes can be made out of a cardboard carton. An oval oven dish makes a serviceable bed pan for the patient who is able only to lie on her side, and a small plastic pail makes an excellent place for an old man to pass water. This can easily be done as the old man sits on the side of his bed holding the pail handle with one hand.

Here is a list of some of the things which a pupil nurse (accompanying the District Nurse) can do in the course of her visit to the home of a sick old person.

The Patient

1 Talk to him and listen to him, don't let the relatives do the talking for him. Find out how he is feeling and what are his needs, and whether he is rational or confused, cheerful or depressed

2 Check temperature, pulse and respiration if necessary

3 Examine the tongue and check that fluid intake is adequate. If not impress the importance of this, arrange that suitable fluids which the patient likes to drink are available, that he can reach them and drink them, and if not that someone is available to do this for him
Ask the patient or relative to record fluid intake, giving guidance as to measures eg an ordinary teacup contains 150ml

4 Enquire about micturition, urine output, continence. If in doubt test urine for sugar and report to general practitioner

5 Check bowels, enquire about diarrhoea, constipation, if necessary examine the rectum

6 Examine the skin, especially pressure points, sacrum, buttocks, trochanters and heels.

7 Examine the limbs for undue muscle wasting and contractures

8 Check finger and toe nails

9 If patient is allowed up check his ability to rise, transfer, stand, walk. Enquire about falls

10 Enquire about diet, ensure that correct ammount of appropriate food is being given and actually consumed by the patient

11 Enquire about sleep, disturbance of others, use of hypnotic drugs

12 Check state of dentures, hearing aids, spectacles, walking sticks or frames, wheelchairs etc

13 Check drugs, ensure that they are accurately labelled and are being taken correctly. Recover drugs no longer required and return to pharmacist

14 Enquire about and encourage leisure interests

15 Carry out necessary procedures, eg injections, enemas, bed bath

16 Prepare report

The Relatives

1 Talk and listen to relatives. Give them an opportunity to talk to you apart from the patient. They may wish to tell you matters that are not for his ears and that can be most informative

2 Check their knowledge of the patient's illness and capabilities. Ensure that they are neither making excessive demands nor are they over protecting him

3 Check their knowledge of patient's drugs

4 Advise on diet, clothing, activities

5 Advise on utilization of other services

6 Enquire what relief family members obtain from their duties

The Environment

1 Check suitability of furniture and floor coverings, advise if necessary

2 Check safety of gas, electric appliances. Report to social worker if in doubt

3 Observe staircase, access to toilet, access to garden or street. Report to Health Visitor if modifications are required

4 Study communications — telephone, warning bell, contact with neighbours, availability and location of door keys

As this by no means comprehensive list indicates, the nurse's role in the home embraces much more than the hospital-based nurse understands by the word 'nursing'. This is what gives the work its added interest. Patients and their relatives turn to the nurse for help, trusting implicitly in her uniform and its traditions and she should be ready to justify their trust in her.

19
Services for the Elderly in the Community

Many an old person languishes at home for want of a service which is available merely because he has never been told that it exists. A nurse can help her patient by making herself familiar with the services available in her own neighbourhood.

In the United Kingdom a whole range of services is provided for old people by Central Government, Local Government and Voluntary Organizations. Essentially similar services are available in many other countries, although there are differences in emphasis and in organization between one area and another. It is useful for the nurse to know something of these services and she can learn more through the medical social worker.

This chapter describes some of the services available for the elderly in the United Kingdom in 1970 but omits organizational details and does not specifically mention the many voluntary organizations which contribute so valuably.

Finance

This is the responsibility of Central Government. It consists of Retirement Pension and Supplementary Benefit.

Retirement Pension

This is paid to men who retire from full-time employment and who have fulfilled certain contributory requirements; also to women who retire and to the widow of an insured person.

The pension is increased if the worker continues in full time employment beyond the normal retirement age, although payment is delayed until he actually retires. It is also increased by graded superannuation contributions.

Supplementary Benefit

This is payable to old people in a wide variety of circumstances and it is very often with enquiry for an application form that a confidential interview can be held to determine the person's eligibility. Supplementary benefits can help old people with their expenses of rent, heating, special diets, domestic help and in other ways. Supplementary Benefit is not a form of charity but is given to those in need as a right to which they have contributed in taxation throughout their working life.

Financial Concessions

Concessions available to pensioners include reduced charges for drugs, transport, public baths, hairdressers, places of entertainment education and many other facilities. Details are available at local Post Offices.

Housing

This is the responsibility of local authorities who in many areas, provide houses specially designed for old people. The earlier blocks of old person's flats are now being replaced by warden service flatlets. The feature of this scheme is that a group of little self-contained flats — usually about 12 to 20 units — is linked to the house of the warden. Each old person has his own front door, pays his own rent and usually prepares his own food, but the warden is there to help him in any difficulties. The warden will see to repairs, call in the doctor, collect pensions or prescriptions, write or telephone to relatives, arrange for the home help to come and so on. The warden can be contacted by a special communication system. Some flatlets schemes have a common room, some provide at least one cooked meal a day; all are centrally heated; some provide additional services like washing machines.

   Similar provision has been made by Housing Associations and other voluntary bodies.

Residential Homes

These are provided by local authorities and voluntary organizations for the benefit of those people who are unable to look after themselves satisfactorily in their own homes, but who do not require nursing attention. Applicants for these homes are expected to be able to wash themselves, dress themselves, attend to their own toilet needs, and to require no human assistance in order to move about within the home. They should by preference be mentally normal but some homes are prepared to accept residents with a degree of mental impairment provided that they present no behaviour problems. There is usually a staff of day and night attendants to help look after the residents.

Homes vary in their structure. A few are still old Poor Houses modernized as much as possible; some are in large villas which have been converted; more and more are 'purpose built'. Residents pay for their accommodation on a sliding scale based on their income. In the modern homes they sleep in single or double bedrooms and they have various lounges, a dining room and a programme of activities to keep them busy and interested. Most of the applicants are very old, the average age on admision being about 80 — a majority are single persons or childless widows or widowers and they are a frail group of people. Medical services are provided by the resident's own general practitioner.

Domiciliary Services

A range of services is available to old people in their own homes. Domestic help is provided by the *Home Help* service of the local authority and in some places by voluntary organizations. The Home Help attends for usually 2 to 4 hours daily and does housework, tidying and cleaning. She may also prepare and serve a meal, shop, collect the pension or a prescription. She is not expected to carry out any nursing tasks. The old person is charged for the service on a scale which takes into account income and family circumstances.

Meals on Wheels

This is a mobile service, provided by the local authority in association with voluntary bodies, which brings hot cooked meals to the homes of old people. A modest charge is made. Old people can also obtain subsidized meals at *luncheon clubs* where the meal is served at some central point such as a Church hall.

Medical and Other Services

Old people in the United Kingdom receive free medical attention from their family doctors and are exempt from the prescription charge. They are also entitled to free dental and ophthalmic treatment and they can be provided with spectacles, dentures and hearing aids and a number of other appliances without charge.

Courses of physiotherapy and occupational therapy can be organised for them free of charge in their own homes, usually on the recommendation of a specialist. Chiropody is also available at a small charge.

Nursing Services

Home nursing is provided by District Nurses who come to the patient daily or less or more often according to need and give a wide range of services such as bathing, application of dressings, injections enemas etc. Health Visitors give advice on health, diet, exercise, and self-care and seek out those old people with medical and social needs and put them in touch with other services. Social workers also act in an advisory role.

There is in the United Kingdom, a trend towards co-ordination of all these services through the establishment of Health Centres where a community nursing team works in close collaboration with family doctors, social workers and visting specialists.

Other Services

Old People's Clubs include those open on one day a week only and those open all day every day, also known as Day Centres. These offer a very wide range of social, cultural, educational, recreational and advisory activities and may also be a means of keeping their members in touch with the health and social services.

Good Neighbours service helps housebound persons by periodic calls on them to see that they are all right and by providing meals, going errands and keeping in touch.

Holidays for old people can be arranged on favourable terms through special agencies.

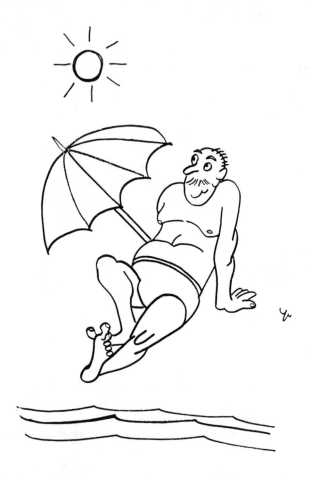

20
Furnishing and Equipment

Nursing the geriatric patient is never easy. Well designed equipment properly serviced and intelligently used can do much to reduce the difficulties. On the other hand poorly conceived and faulty items of equipment which are wrongly used, can add greatly to the nurse's difficulties.

Because the equipment used in different hospitals varies so much this chapter will be concerned with the general principles of design, use and maintenance. Physiotherapy equipment is not dealt with.

Beds

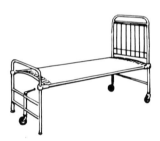

Ordinary Bed with Lock

The simplest hospital bed is a metal frame — approximately 2 metres long, just under 1 metre wide, and 58 cm high. The modern hospital bed is a sophisticated piece of machinery with many attachments and refinements which make the bed more comfortable for the patient and facilitate the nurse's work.

Here are some features of the modern bed:

Wheels — Ease of movement of the bed is necessary for cleaning floors and for moving bed patients from one area to another. Wheels need brakes, otherwise an accident may occur if the patient leans against the bed and it rolls away from him. If these are foot-operated the action must be easy, the hold firm, and the brake should be clearly marked so that it is apparent at a glance whether the brake is applied or not.

Base of Bed
This can either be spring or solid wood perforated for ventilation. The latter is more suitable for modern light-weight foam mattresses.

Stripper
This may either fold down or pull out from the foot of the bed. It should be broad enough to support all the covers during bed making. Metal is preferable to formica which has a slippery surface.

Back Rest

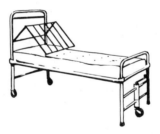

Adjustable Back Rest

This should be infinitely variable in position. The catch to alter the position should be operated readily with the use of one hand.

Detachable Head and Foot
These fittings are useful when lifting a heavy or unconscious patient from bed to trolley.

Cot Sides

These should be easy to erect, fasten securely, should remain attached to the bed when not in use — either folded down or slid underneath. The bars should be so spaced that a patient with a small head cannot get it stuck between the bars!

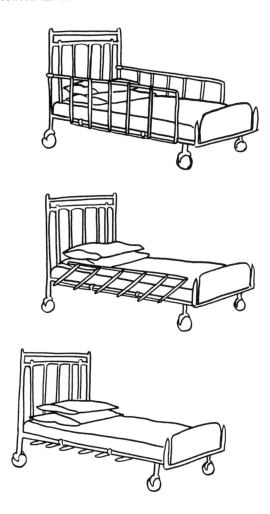

Lifting Pole

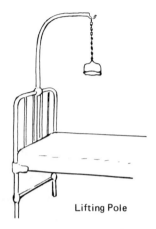

Lifting Pole

This lifting pole is usually at the head of the bed. A model is also available which attaches to the side of the bed.

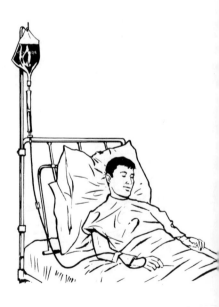

Drip-Stand Attachment

This is of particular advantage when patients are moved to theatre, x-ray department, etc in their beds with an infusion running.

The Variable Height Bed
The standard hospital bed is at a suitable height for bed-making and for carrying out nursing procedures for a patient in bed. But it is too high for many patients to get in and out of bed comfortably.

The variable height bed has many advantages for the geriatric patient and for his nurse.

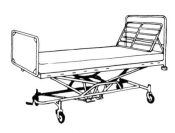

Variable Height Bed

At the low height it facilitates the rehabilitation of patients going home to a low divan bed. The danger of the patient falling when getting up during the night is lessened if his feet touch the floor immediately he puts his legs over the side of the bed.

The variable bed can be raised to a height of 66 cm or lowered to a height of 45 cm. The variable height mechanism can be operated manually by turning a handle as shown in model illustrated; hydraulically by operating a foot pump; or electrically by pressing a button.

Variable Position Bed
The mechanism allows the head of the bed to be raised while the foot is lowered; or vice versa. In more complicated beds the base is divided into three sections which can be moved separately or together to give a variety of positions.

Bed Cages
These are designed to take the weight of the bed clothes off the patient' feet. They can be inserted under the mattress at the foot or side of the bed. A cage which stands inside the bed can ease pressure on the patients feet (see pages 21 and 116).

Bed Head Fittings
These include a reading light, a radio receiver with earphones and a nurse call system. The controls for these devices should be clearly distinguished from one another and their use explained to the patient. All should be available to the bed patient without his having to perform acrobatic feats.

Mattresses
These can be spring-interior or light weight triple foam — 10 cm deep. The mattress should be protected by a waterproof cover. The more modern nylon type of mattress cover does not seem to cause excessive heating of the skin.

Sheets
Cotton sheets remain the most satisfactory for hospital use. They are cool to the patient's skin and are easily laundered by hospital laundries.

Blankets
Cellular wool or cotton are light weight and are easily washed — a property appreciated more by nurses than by patients.

Continental Quilts — 'Downies'
A continental type quilt covering facilitates bed-making and is light weight yet warm for the patient. It is suitable for many patients but not for the frequently incontinent.

Pillows
Traditional down pillows are easily moulded to the desired position. Foam pillows are lighter and (theoretically) safer since the patient can breathe through them, but more rigid.

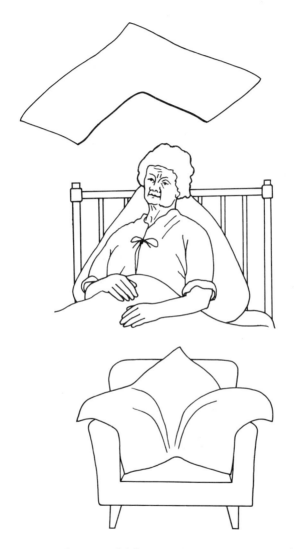

The Wundarest pillow is useful for propping up patients in a chair or in bed. It is equally useful at home or in hospital.

Variable Pressure Mattresses

There are a group of mechanically operated mattresses used in addition to the ordinary mattress in an attempt to vary the distribution of pressure over the trunk of the immobile patient, and so reduce the danger of pressure sores.

The Ripple Bed

The alternating pressure mattress or *ripple bed* – is made of stout plastic material and is placed on top of the mattress and covered by a sheet. It is divided either longitudinally or transversely into a number of air cells, which vary in width in different models from 4 cm to 15 cm. The larger cell varieties are preferable. The mattress is attached to an air pump which inflates alternate cells and simultaneously deflates those lying between, so that part of the patient's body is raised off the bed. Every 15 minutes or so the cycle alternates, so that the formerly inflated cells are deflated and vice versa, and a different part of the patient's body is then protected from pressure. This device can make a very useful contribution to the prevention of pressure sores. It is usually quite well tolerated by patients on the whole. The principal troubles are puncture of the air cells with loss of pressure and mechanical breakdown of the pump. Sometimes failure of the instrument to operate is merely due to a tube having become disconnected.

Variable Pressure Control

Some models have a variable pressure control or at least a change of high and low pressure, selection of the appropriate pressure being determined by the weight of the patient. Nurses should check the performance of the alternating pressure mattress by ensuring that cells are inflating and deflating properly and that the patient's body is being lifted clear of the deflated cells (see page 128).

Pneumatic Mattress

This operates on a rather similar principle but consist only of two longitudinal cells which are placed under the mattress inflating and deflating alternately in a 15-minute cycle and they have the effect of lifting the patient from side to side, thus transferring the patient's weight from one part of the body to another. The distance apart of the two cells can be adjusted according to the weight of the patient. The closer together they are placed the steeper is the angle of tilt. This mattress is effective and well tolerated. The cells are made of stout plastic and are unlikely to puncture.

Lockers

There are probably more different types of bedside locker on the market than of any other piece of hospital equipment, indicating the difficulty of designing one to suit all possible uses. Selection of a suitable locker depends on the clarity with which the purchaser considers the questions: — 'What do I want to use it for'? The essential requirements are:

1 A top surface accessible to the patient in bed on which can be rested safely and without fear of spillage a tumbler, a jug of water, bottles of soft drinks. There should also be a space for a sputum cup. An easily wiped surface and a raised edge are essential

2 An easily opened compartment directly accessible to the patient from either side of the bed is required for storage of money, spectacles, cigarettes, paper tissues and cosmetics

3 A partly concealed compartment for a urinal is an advantage

4 The remaining space is available for slippers, bed jacket, dressing gown (possibly) reading and writing materials, food extras etc. This area is not safely reached from bed and should be opened by the nurse

5 There is a rail for towel and toilet bag

The locker should be light so that it can be mobile to facilitate cleaning. Castors may be dangerous as the patient may tend to lean on the locker and braking is not practical.

Articles which it is not convenient to put on or in a locker include vases of flowers and patient's outer clothing and shoes and soiled linen. Combined lockers and clothing cupboards are available but they take up a lot of space around the bed and separate wardrobes against the wall are preferable.

Lockers with hinged tray attachments are very suitable in conjunction with variable height beds and do away with the need for a separate over bed table.

Overbed Tables

These may be of cantilever or bridge type, the latter having wheels or skids. The cantilever type take up less space, are easy to move and are variable in height, but some makes are too small, so that the patient has to sit sideways to reach the table. The bridge type are usually of fixed height and can then be uncomfortable for the patient, but variable height models are available. They are difficult to use in conjunction with cot sides or foot cages. Some models have a panel which slides up to give a reading stand.

Adjustable Bed Table

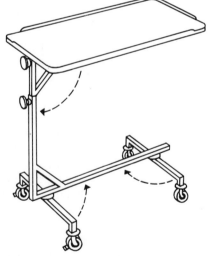

This table has adjustable height mechanism and folds flat for easy storage.

Chairs

The ideal chair for the geriatric patient has not yet been invented nor is it ever likely to be, because we require so many properties of a chair, but clever adaptations to chairs can be made. Geriatric wards should have a number of different types of chair to meet a variety of needs, the main common factor is that they must have arms. The right chair will be selected if the nurse asks herself 'What do I want this chair to do for this patient?'.

Here are some of the attributes of a good chair:

1 Stability
2 Ease of getting out
3 Comfort
4 Mobility
5 Ease of cleaning
6 Space

Stability

The chair must not tip over when the patient exerts pressure on rising or sitting down firmly. This requires that the legs be splayed out to some in front of and behind the seat. Since hemiplegic patients tend to press down on one arm of the chair only on rising a chair used by them should also have its leg splayed out to the side. The legs should be covered by a rubber ferrule to prevent the chair slipping.

2 Ease of Getting Out

For ease of rising a chair must have a firm, level high seat — a height of at least 35 cm being required. There must be no bar between the front legs which might prevent the patient from placing his feet back on rising and the arms should be low in front to give maximum purchase.

Any chair can be made easier to get out of by a firm cushion or by use of a special spring device placed on top of the seat.

3 Comfort

Comfort is dependent on good design more than on soft upholstery.

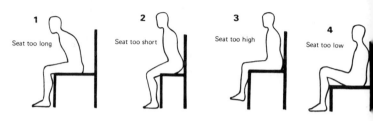

The necessary features are a level seat moulded to the shape of the buttocks, a space between the seat and the back to accommodate the patient's bottom, and enable him to sit well back into the chair; a moulded back which supports the small of the patient's back and padded arms. (See page 24)

4 Mobility

If the patient is to be moved in his chair an arrangement of wheels and brakes is necessary. It is difficult to design this in a manner which is safe and comfortable (although some fairly good attempts have been made) without resorting to a wheelchair. Such an arrangement is necessary only for helpless patients who are lifted out of bed into the chair, then moved in it to the day room, thus reducing the number of transfers required. Any ordinary chair can be converted into a mobile chair by the addition of castors. A special device is available which can be connected in a moment under any chair to transform it into a wheelchair.

6 Ease of Cleansing

The surface should be of plastic or other water-repellent material for ease of cleansing and wiping down and it should be able to resist urine.

6 Space

Consideration should be given to the amount of space which the chair occupies and to whether it can be stacked.

Wheelchairs

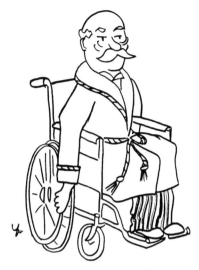

Self-propelled wheelchairs are of great use and many patients require no other type of chair, finding them quite comfortable and being able to get into and out of them without great difficulty. The main points to look for in a wheelchair are as follows:

1 Stability
2 Mobility
3 Foot plates
4 Attachments

1 Stability

A wheelchair is inevitably less stable than an ordinary chair and the patient must be skilful at sitting down gently before using a wheelchair. The brakes can be difficult to operate, especially to put into the fully on position. Some geriatric patients require frequent reminders to check that their brakes are on.

2 Mobility

If the tyres are not solid they must be properly inflated, otherwise driving becomes very difficult. The small swivel front wheels are difficult to control on an uneven surface or on a carpet and the patient must use quite a lot of strength.

3 Foot Plates
These are difficult to operate and may cause a nasty blow on the shins.

4 Attachments
The standard chair may be modified by having straight leg attachments, removable sides, commode attachments, extended brake levers.

Commodes

Modern nursing practice is to bring the commode to the patient's bedside, to use a disposable bed pan in it, to transfer the patient from bed to commode and back again, to remove the commode back to its storage area, to remove the bedpan and dispose of it and to wipe down the seat. These requirements determine the design of the modern commode and it must combine mobility with stability, be easy to get on and off, be easily stored and easily wiped down and have a suitable shelf on which the bedpan is placed.

Sanitary chairs

These consist of a frame and a toilet seat. The patient sits on the chair which is taken to the lavatory and wheeled over the water closet. These are of value when the space in the toilet is too restricted to enable the patient to be transferred from wheelchair to the lavatory and when he is unable to use a commode. They avoid the need for disposing of a bedpan but on the other hand they occupy a lot of space. They are not convenient when the toilet is distant.

Toilets

The time and thought given by an architect to the design of the toilet area and the selection of equipment can do more to increase or diminish the work of the nurses than any other design which he makes in building a hospital. Some of the difficulties which arise are due to conflicting requirements.

Door

The doorway must be wide enough to allow a wheelchair to pass in comfort ie 84 cm. This means a big heavy door which occupies a lot of space in the toilet, and round which the chair must be manoeuvered.

There are several solutions.

1 Making the door open outwards (disliked by architects because of danger to passers-by)

2 Splitting the door

3 Replacing the door by a plastic curtain

4 Providing a sliding door

5 Enlarging the toilet area

The lavatory pan is usually placed in the middle of the back wall with no room for the wheelchair or sanitary chair to be placed at right angles to the pan so as to allow an easy transfer.

Nurses often have to clamber over the chair once it gets into the toilet and have then to do a transfer in a far from ideal position.

Hand Rails

Hand rails beside the toilet are of great value in helping the patient to sit down and rise again. These may be fixed to the walls, bolted to the floor or (less satisfactorily) moved in and placed on the floor. An excellent variety is fixed to the wall behind the toilet and can be slid down for use. Vertical poles, ropes and all kinds of hand grips can also be used, but use of the toilet roll fixture as a hand grip should be discouraged.

Raised Toilet Seats

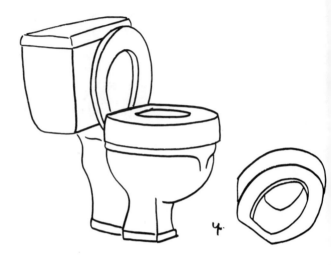

These are very helpful, and are made of wood or polypropylene in different sizes and are simply placed over the toilet seat.

Toilet Roll Dispensers
Individual sheets are easier for hemiplegic patients than tear off rolls.

Bedpans and Urinals
Disposable bedpans are now widely used in conjunction with machines, which generaly operate satisfactorily provided that the manufacturers instructions are strictly adhered to. Mechanical breakdown is most frustrating and good maintenance and repair arrangements must be made.

21
Day Room Activities

The word activity does not necessarily mean actual physical activity — it means in this context either mental or physical activity which will interest the elderly person, encourage him to try to do new things, and make purposeful use of the time on his hands.

Simplicity should be the keynote of the activities and indeed the materials they use should be clean and any tools should be as safe as possible.

Many older people will enjoy knitting and while a garment, scarf, or pair of socks would be too long a knit for them they would be glad to knit squares for blankets — particularly if the blankets were destined for the maternity or children's wards of the hospital. Although wool is expensive to buy — it is usually only necessary to mention the need to a Church Guild, Girl Guides, or some of the Voluntary Services and the supplies are forthcoming.

The following are suggestions which you may find useful:

Seasonal Activities

Christmas provides an abundance of excuses for activity. Decorations, Christmas Cards, Calendars, can all be made.

Plain serviettes can be suitably decorated. Attractive table centres can be made with pieces of holly, a candle, a metal foil dish and some plaster of paris.

Invitations to various parties, or functions provide another activity.

Social Activities

It is not always desirable to have activities which the person does alone.

Social activities are very important and various simple card games, Dominoes, Bingo, Skittles etc can raise quite a bit of fun.

Music is also a useful aid and indeed a percussion band is noisy but fun. Old people like to sing 'their' songs and the wise nurse will have a list of these somewhere in the duty room as when she sits down at the piano her mind becomes a complete blank!! The key and the starting note is a useful bit of information to write alongside the name of the song!

Notable events on Television can be highlighted.

Caring for a ward budgie is another way of 'employing' someone's spare time.

There is also a visit from an outsider to show coloured films or slides and improbable as it may be many geriatric units have had demonstration of flower arrangement, hat making, etc. A conjuror can pass a weary winter hour with them.

Celebrities too are usually most helpful about coming to the hospital.

Groups of youngsters also can come occasionally carol-singing etc. Old people have a special communication with young people and are delighted to have visits from them.

The children from a local Nursery can also visit the ward and even if the visit is brief the old people get interest in watching the toddlers and indeed in seeing their progress from time to time.

A tropical fish tank is an attractive focal point.

Outings of any kind are to be encouraged.

Window boxes — indoor and outdoor can provide endless interest and pleasure for some old people.

Remember too to include if you can some form of religious worship. This may only be a question of hymn singing or possibly a visit occasionally from a section of a church choir.

But while these activities are mostly involving noise — remember some old people like to sit quietly looking at a magazine through photographs, quietly chatting to visitors or each other — so be sure to have some quiet corner away from the bustle for them.

An elderly person in hospital enjoys getting mail and it is up to the ward personnel to try and encourage this.

One ward had a large book and in it the dates of the birthdays of several of each patient's relatives. Nurse saw to it that a card went to the

180

relative concerned around the correct date and of course a letter came back in reply.

Some old person may like to polish brass or silver — why not have a few pieces in the Day Room for her to polish?

22
On Being Old

These thoughts were written by a lady of seventy-eight.

A patient's views on being old

Difficulties like losing sight and hearing and inability to get into baths etc because of diminishing agility are easier to put up with than smaller common ones like:

1 Difficulties in fastening clothes — buttons, studs, bras, shoes, zips

2 General clumsiness — dropping tickets, pencils, money

3 Difficulty in understanding instructions, directions, some conversations, jokes, and the filling in of forms

4 The allround slowing down of tempo in every day life takes time to get used to — in and out of the house

5 The fact that favourite foods no longer taste so good

6 The surroundings you live with are getting more and more worn and when a repair is needed it seems to take so much effort to do

7 Threading a needle becomes an effort, and sewing slow and difficult

8 The inability of public transport officials to understand that you cannot nip on and off buses like a young one

9 The recurring and inevitable news of friends dying on certain days has a very depressing influence

10 The wireless becomes a greater companion than television very often as it seems to be a more personal thing and it is easier just to hear than to watch and hear at the same time as you do in television although it is lovely to watch the sort of pagentry things on television.

11 It is difficult to accept that your children are mature adults and may be capable of advising you what to do

12 It is delightful to be helped in a courteous and gracious way but just awful when you feel it is being done in a patronising way.

Elizabeth A.

23
Further Reading

AGATE, J. (1972)
Geriatrics for Nurses and Social Workers
Heinemann Medical Books, London

EDMONDSON, E. (1971)
Nursing the Incontinent
Butterworths, London

EXTON-SMITH, A. N., NORTON, D., McLAREN, R. (1962)
An Investigation of Geriatric Nursing Problems in Hospital
National Corporation for the Care of Old People, London

FRANCIS, G. (1973)
Caring for the Elderly
Heinemann Medical Books, London

IRVINE, R. E., BAGNALL, M. K., SMITH, B. J. (1970)
The Older Patient
English Universities Press

ISAACS, B. (1965)
An Introduction to Geriatrics
Bailliere, Tindall and Cassell, London

RUDD, T. M. (1967)
Human Relations in Old Age
Faber and Faber, London

THOMSON, M. K. (1969)
Geriatrics and the General Practitioner Team
Bailliere, Tindall and Cassell, London
Equipment for the Disabled
The National Fund for Research into Crippling Disease

WALKER, K. A. (1971)
Pressure Sores, Prevention and Treatment
Butterworths, London

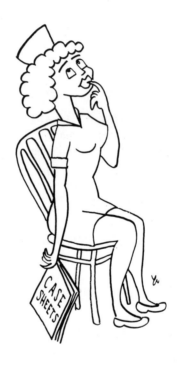

Index